AMERICAN JOURNAL of PUBLIC HEALTH
DECEMBER 2023
Issue 12

AJPH

A PUBLICATION OF THE
AMERICAN PUBLIC HEALTH ASSOCIATION

TOWARD MORE EQUITABLE PUBLIC HEALTH DATA

Insights and Examples, p. 1276
Gaps and Opportunities, p. 1301
Federal Agencies, p. 1278
NHANES and Medi-Cal, pp. 1283 and 1290
Sexual and Gender Minority, p. 1287
Asian American, Native Hawaiian, and Pacific Islander, p. 1296

Also in this issue:

FIREARM SUICIDE AND HOMICIDE
New York SAFE Act, 1999–2019, pp. 1238 and 1309

HIGH-CONCENTRATION CANNABIS
Review of Health Effects, p. 1332

ABORTION
Among US Incarcerated Persons, p. 1352

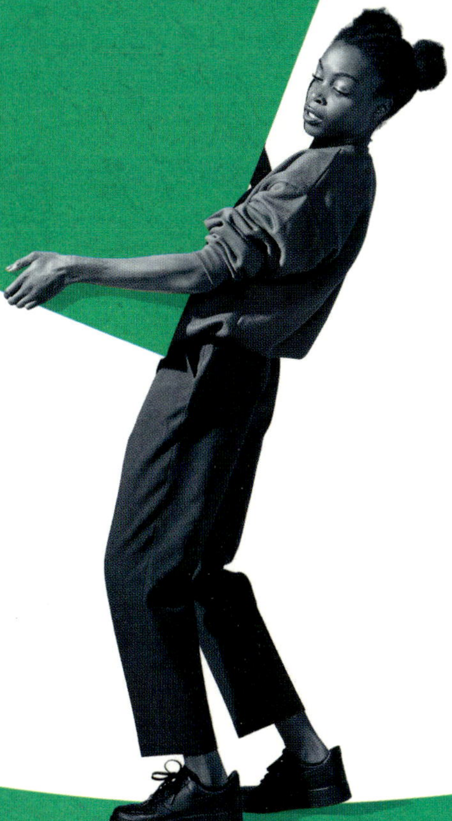

AMERICAN PUBLIC HEALTH ASSOCIATION
For science. For action. For health.

AJPH®, published monthly, is the official Journal of the American Public Health Association®, 800 I St NW, Washington, DC 20001-3710; (202) 777- APHA; TDD (202) 777-2500. APHA is a nongovernmental professional society founded in 1872, representing all disciplines and specialties in public health.

The *American Journal of Public Health*® (*AJPH*) (print ISSN: 0090-0036; electronic ISSN: 1541- 0048), first published in 1911, is the official journal of the American Public Health Association® (APHA). The oldest and largest organization of public health professionals in the world, APHA represents approximately 30 000 members from more than 50 occupations of public health.

Submissions: Visit www.editorialmanager.com/ajph or ajph.edmgr.com for online manuscript preparation and submission guidelines. Contributions of original unpublished research, social science analyses, scholarly essays, critical commentaries, departments, and letters to the editor are welcome. Questions? Write ajph.submissions@apha.org or call APHA at (202) 777-2469.

Print plus online subscriptions: Institutional price (print copy with online access for a single institution and all authorized users, regardless of geographic location) varies by size of organization and ranges from $993–$1445 for US organizations, and $1073–$1526 for international organizations (air delivery); multiple campuses not permitted without special arrangement. Details of the tiered pricing system at https://subscriptionoffice.com/pages/apha-landing-page. To order, write apha.subscriptions@apha.org.

Online-only subscriptions: Institutional price for one institution and its authorized users (regardless of geographic location) is $878–$1307. To order, write apha.subscriptions@apha.org. For academic consortia or multisite corporate subscriptions, contact apha.subscriptions@apha.org.

Print-only subscriptions: Institutional price is US $701, $782 international.

Back print issues: A limited number of print issues are for sale. Single copies are US $49, $55 international (air delivery). Shipping included; prepay only. To order, write apha.subscriptions@apha.org.

Reprints: For prices and ordering information on 50 or more reprints, check the Reprints section at www.ajph.org. To order smaller quantities of reprints (rush delivery), use the "Purchase Article" link on the article site itself.

Electronic access: Online articles more than 10 years old are available free for personal use at www.ajph.org. Recent articles are available through pay-per-view: single PDF article for $24, single issue access for 24 hours for $33, or entire site access for 24 hours for $38.

Postal information: Periodicals postage paid at Washington, DC, and additional mailing offices. Postmaster: Send address changes to American Journal of Public Health, 800 I St NW, Washington, DC 20001-3710.

Address changes: Send to AJPH, Membership Department (members) or AJPH Subscriptions (subscribers), APHA, 800 I St NW, Washington, DC 20001-3710. Or write to membership.mail@apha. org (members) or apha.subscriptions@apha.org (subscribers).

Advertising: For pricing and other information, see www.ajph.org. Please write to ashell.alston@apha.org or call (202) 777-2470 for other advertising opportunities. Ask about special exhibit packages and sponsorships. Acceptance of advertising by the *Journal* does not imply endorsement of products.

Indexes: Publications that index or abstract articles from AJPH include the following: Ageline, Assia (Applied Social Science Index and Abstracts), Biological Abstracts, Chemical Abstracts, CINAHL, Criminal Justice Abstracts, EMBASE, EMCare, Environmental Abstracts, e-psyche, ERIC, ETOH (Alcohol and Alcohol Problems Science Database), Excerpta Medica, Food Science and Technology, General Science Index, Grateful Med, Hospital Literature Index, Human Resources Abstracts, International Pharmaceutical Abstracts (IPA), Medline, Physical Education Index, Pollution Abstracts, Psychological Abstracts, PsychINFO, Safety Science Abstracts, Sage Family Studies Abstracts, Sage Human Resources Abstracts, Science Citation Index, SCOPUS, SIIC Data Bases, Social Work Research and Abstracts, and Statistical Reference Index (SRI)/LexisNexis.

AJPH

A PUBLICATION OF THE
AMERICAN PUBLIC HEALTH ASSOCIATION

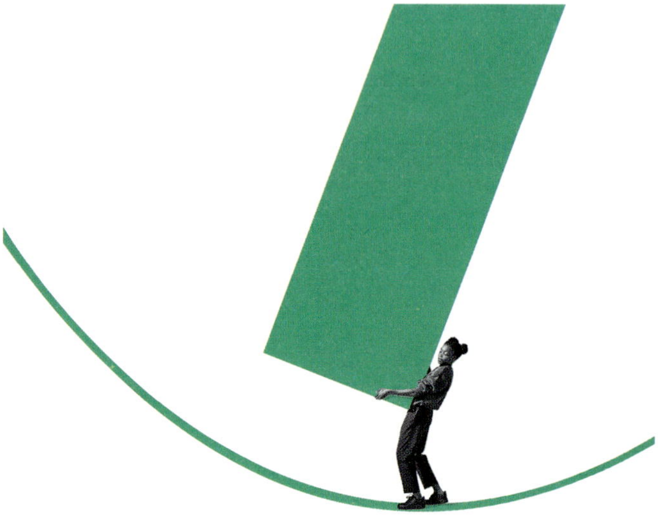

COVER: To transform the data narrative, there must be purposeful efforts toward creating better data content, processes, and infrastructures that do not mask systemic inequities. We hope this special issue inspires action and spurs progress toward achieving data systems that track existing inequities in public health.

Cover concept and selection by Aleisha Kropf, Image Editor. Image by Klaus Vedfelt/Getty Images. Printed with permission.

APHA
AMERICAN PUBLIC HEALTH ASSOCIATION
For science. For action. For health.

Promoting public health research, policy, practice, and education is the *AJPH* mission. As we widen our scope to embrace global issues, we also sharpen our focus to support the needs of public health practitioners. We invite contributions of original unpublished research, opinion and commentary, and letters to the editor.

The *Journal* is printed on acid-free recycled paper.

AJPH December 2023, Vol 113, No. 12

OPEN ACCESS ONLINE ONLY PODCAST DATA SUPPLEMENT AVAILABLE

EDITOR'S CHOICE

1237 Play, Read, and Vote for Health
C. Chanyasulkit

OPINIONS, IDEAS, & PRACTICE

EDITORIALS

1238 Supporting Multicomponent Gun Control Laws: A Need for Valid and Comprehensive Research
E. Blais

1241 From *Roe* to *Dobbs*: The Critical Role of Medical Housing for Individuals Seeking Abortion Care
J. A. Owens, F. R. W. Lilly, A. Allen, M. Falcon, and R. J. Ward

PERSPECTIVES

1244 Overcoming Barriers to Training the Next Generation of Public Health Professionals
S. Z. Nasruddin, T. Johnson, M. Presley, B. Wade, Q. Whalen, E. Gordineer, C. Compretta, E. Dehon, A. Ford-Wade, M. Godfrey, and M. Barnard

1249 Typhoid Mary Was Not a Super-Spreader (and Super-Spreaders Are Not "Typhoid Marys")
A. Teicher

NOTES FROM THE FIELD

1254 A Medicaid-Funded Statewide Diabetes Quality Improvement Collaborative: Ohio 2020–2022
S. D. Bolen, J. J. Joseph, K. M. Dungan, E. A. Beverly, A. T. Perzynski, D. Einstadter, J. Fiegl, T. E. Love, D. Spence, K. Jenkins, A. Lorenz, S. J. Uddin, K. McCutcheon Adams, M. W. Konstan, and M. S. Applegate, on behalf of the Diabetes Quality Improvement Collaborative

1258 Countering Mpox Vaccination Disparities in Los Angeles County, California, May–December 2022
A. Brihn, N. Yeganeh, S. Kulkarni, O. Moir, S. Madrid, M. Perez, R. Singhal, and A. A. Kim

1263 Reversing Inequity in Mpox Vaccine Distribution, Fulton County, Georgia, June–September 2022
J. O'Neal, J. Lopes da Rosa, M. Astin, D. Folkes, D. Crowder, and D. P. Holland

1267 Evaluating e-Connect: Mitigating Race by Gender Disparities in Behavioral Health Referral Among Youths on Probation, Northeast United States, 2019
M. E. Ryan, K. S. Elkington, C. Sarapas, C. Sichel, F. Taxman, M. L. Dennis, and G. A. Wasserman

1271 Child Safety Seat–Use Behavior Among Parents of Newborns: A Trans-Theoretical Model–Guided Intervention in Shantou, China, 2021
Y. Peng, F. Wu, J. Yang, and L. Li

TOWARD MORE EQUITABLE PUBLIC HEALTH DATA

1276 Toward More Equitable Public Health Data: An *AJPH* Special Section
N. A. Ponce and D. T. Lau

1278 The Federal Agencies' Hidden Efforts to Produce Equitable Data
A. O'Hara and R. Rhodes

1283 Medi-Cal's Population Health Management Program: Advancing Shared Medicaid and Public Health Data Processes and Infrastructure
S. Sharma, P. Babaria, D. Tian, and L. Scott

1287 Advancing Sexual and Gender Minority Population Health Using Electronic Health Record Data
K. E. Baker, E. Sarkodie, J. Kwait, C. Medina, A. Radix, and R. Flynn

1290 Data Related to Social Determinants of Health Captured in the National Health and Nutrition Examination Survey
D. T. Lau, N. Ahluwalia, C. D. Fryar, M. Kaufman, I. E. Arispe, and R. Paulose-Ram

1296 Championing the 2021 New York State Law: A Step Toward Data Disaggregation on Asian Americans, Native Hawaiians, and Pacific Islanders
A. Gundanna, C. M. Calhoon, M. Anand, L. Feng, and V. Leung

RESEARCH & ANALYSIS

TOWARD MORE EQUITABLE PUBLIC HEALTH DATA

1301 Social Determinants of Health, Quality of Public Health Data, and Health Equity in the United States
S. H. Sheingold, R. B. Zuckerman, N. De Lew, and A. Chappel

OPEN-THEMED RESEARCH

1309 Association Between the New York SAFE Act and Firearm Suicide and Homicide: An Analysis of Synthetic Controls, New York State, 1999–2019
I. M. Karaye, G. Knight, and C. Kyriacou

1318 Child Mental Health Status in Flint, Michigan: A Worsening Health Inequity, 2018–2022
J. Dannis, S. Jenuwine, N. Jones, J. LaChance, and M. Hanna-Attisha

1322 Employee Cardiometabolic Risk Following a Cluster-Randomized Workplace Intervention From the Work, Family and Health Network, 2009–2013
L. F. Berkman, E. L. Kelly, L. B. Hammer, F. Mierzwa, T. Bodner, T. McNamara, H. K. Koga, S. Lee, M. Marino, L. C. Klein, T. W. McDade, G. Hanson, P. Moen, and O. M. Buxton

1332 Health Effects of High-Concentration Cannabis Products: Scoping Review and Evidence Map
L. Bero, R. Lawrence, J.-P. Oberste, T. Li, L. Leslie, T. Rittiphairoj, C. Piper, G. S. Wang, A. Brooks-Russell, T. W. Yim, G. Tung, and J. M. Samet

1343 Health Disparities Among Sexual and Gender Minorities With Adverse Childhood Experiences: Insights From the 2021 Behavioral Risk Factor Surveillance System Data
M. A. Solberg, L. M. Blair, E. C. Schlegel, and J. A. M. J. Kurzer

1352 Incarceration Status Among Individuals Obtaining Abortion in the United States, 2020
M. Kirstein, L. Fuentes, and C. Sufrin

BACKMATTER

LETTERS & RESPONSES

1356 COVID-19 Experience Reflects the Importance of Understanding the Impacts of Public Health Policies and Long COVID on Pediatric Populations
M. Berger

1357 Connolly and Golden Respond
C. Connolly and J. Golden

OTHER DEPARTMENTS

1360 Subscription Form

Play, Read, and Vote for Health

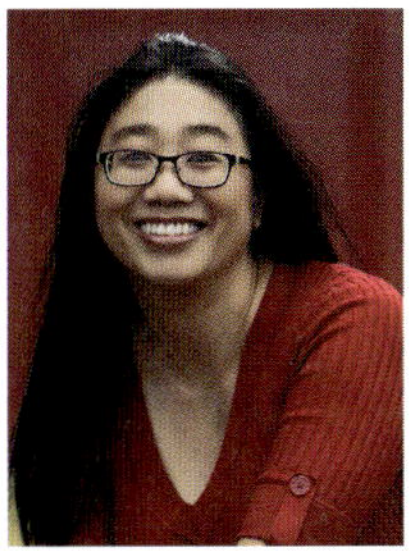

As American Public Health Association president, I've traveled across the nation to visit state public health associations and educational institutions—such as Boise State University, Idaho State University, and the University of Texas Medical Branch in Galveston—and connect with community leaders and students to share my three steps of playing, reading, and voting for a healthier nation.

PLAY

I call on all of us, particularly those who have worked tirelessly in public health during the COVID-19 pandemic, to take a moment each day to play. This is crucial to our mental and physical health and will allow us to continue to do the much-needed good work. Although busy with our work, families, and communities, don't forget to take some time for yourself to reflect, recharge, relax, and find moments of joy.

These can be solo or shared experiences such as taking a walk, doing a puzzle, knitting, or playing a board or online game. My family is big into card and board games! Every day I'm thankful for the opportunity to walk my dogs, Oswald and Dolly, at least a few times a day. Perhaps the greatest lesson that I've learned from them is to be sure to take time outside and "smell the roses." They stop a lot to smell pretty much everything, but it's made a world of difference in my life.

READ

With so much misinformation, disinformation, and censorship and so many book-banning efforts, I want us to get back to more reading, as this is critical for combating misinformation. This reading can be active. We can collaborate and partner with other organizations to share our ideas for healthier communities through op-eds and letters to the editors in local news outlets; local journalism is important and a great community connector. Plus, reading can be fun and a good way to "play" for health too. You can often find me listening to an audiobook while out for a walk with my dogs, when I'm not reading *AJPH* of course. And sometimes, of course, I'm listening to *AJPH* podcasts, too (shameless plug)!

VOTE

It's critical that all eligible voters vote, especially in local and state elections. Every day our local and state governments make important decisions that affect our community health. I believe that to truly make impactful change in the public health and well-being of communities across our nation, participation in local elections is key.

We need to focus on engaging and informing local voters to elect candidates who prioritize public health. Our elected officials need to understand how they play a critical public health role in the laws that they enact. We need them to understand that affordable and safe housing is public health, that access to safe and reliable transportation is public health, and that we don't have a moment to waste on addressing climate change.

Research shows that the majority of our nation supports addressing climate change, the right to abortion, and stronger gun control. Research also shows that many of our state and federal elected officials do not hold these majority views, nor do they govern as most of the nation wants. With this glaring disconnect, I believe that if all eligible voters voted, it would make a world of difference toward making this a healthier and more inclusive world. Again, local elections matter.

With each affiliate visit (to Alaska, New Hampshire, and many places in between), I am heartened to hear the many ways that public health practitioners are sharing their health information with their policymakers and are doing their level best to inform elected officials of the importance of public health for their constituents.

I was thrilled to meet Aditi Bussells, an at-large councilwoman representing Columbia, South Carolina, and to hear her speak at the South Carolina Public Health Association's annual conference about how she brings her education and background in public health to her policymaking. How incredible would it be if every policymaker at every level of government had a grounding in public health?

Perhaps as you read this, you will consider running for office, too! Maybe I need to revise my call to action? "Play, read, and vote (and possibly run) for health."

Finally, as I head into being immediate past president, know that my call to play, read, and vote for health does not end here. It's only just beginning. We need to stay fierce and focused on our mission to create a healthier, more inclusive, and kinder world. Bring this call to play, read, and vote for health to every corner of our precious planet—we don't have a moment to lose. AJPH

Chris Chanyasulkit, PhD, MPH
President
American Public Health Association

DOI: https://doi.org/10.2105/AJPH.2023.307491

50 Years Ago

Desegregating Health Statistics

The separation of American health statistics into basic categories of white and nonwhite is a reflection of our heritage of racial segregation. . . . The white–nonwhite dichotomy is indefensible on scientific grounds, since the groups included in the nonwhite category have widely divergent mortality rates. . . . [S]ome of these groups have lower death rates than whites, while others have higher rates. Why then are they lumped together? The confusion is further compounded by the official designation, within the nonwhite group, of Chinese and Japanese as separate races, a classification which is difficult to comprehend since these are clearly not races but nationalities. The designation of Mexicans as nonwhites in 1932 through 1934 and the change from "race" in the 1900-1940 volume on Vital Statistics Rates in the United States to "color" in the 1940–1960 volume, indicate that the designations and categories are shifting and unstable, reflecting political pressures instead of scientific procedures.

From AJPH, June 1973, p. 478

61 Years Ago

Social Implications Of Race-Color Designations

In the history of vital statistics and public health research, race has been a meaningful category. The differentials between whites and nonwhites in health status and in death rates at birth have been analyzed and the findings employed to develop programs for the improvement of life chances. . . . In view of the advantages of including racial designation as an item on vital records, . . . it is not easy to understand the movement to have this practice discontinued in many geographic areas. . . . [T]he opposition's argument . . . "is that the inclusion of racial designations on personal records violates personal privacy and/or individual rights and may lead to preferential treatment or discriminatory action. . . . The real danger is in having no statistics, rather than in having them as a basis of evaluation. Rumors and prejudice are likely to thrive in those areas which cannot be evaluated. In this connection it can be stated categorically that reliable statistics by race in those areas where discrimination and civil rights violations are alleged afford the minority group the best protection it can hope to have."

From AJPH, April 1962, pp. 671–674.

AJPH December 2023, Vol 113, No. 12

Supporting Multicomponent Gun Control Laws: A Need for Valid and Comprehensive Research

Etienne Blais, PhD

ABOUT THE AUTHOR

Etienne Blais is with the School of Criminology, University of Montreal, Montreal, Quebec, Canada.

See also Karaye et al., p. 1309.

In their article in this issue of *AJPH* (p. 1309), Karaye et al. assessed the impact of the New York Secure Ammunition and Firearms Enforcement Act (NY SAFE Act) on firearm-related suicide and homicide rates for the 1999 to 2019 period.[1] Introduced in January 2013, the NY SAFE Act contains many provisions going beyond the general federal requirements, such as increased background checks before the purchase of a firearm and ammunition, prohibition of large-capacity magazines and some semiautomatic weapons, a red flag system, and safe storage conditions. The authors' results indicated that the NY SAFE Act was associated with a significant decrease in firearm-related homicides, whereas firearm-related suicides were not affected. Furthermore, the authors did not observe any substitution effect. Their findings suggest that multicomponent gun control laws can prevent firearm-related homicides.

Their article has two main contributions: (1) the method they used to estimate the impact of the act, which overcame several threats to internal validity usually found in evaluations of gun control laws, and (2) the implications for future studies and public health policy that emerge from their discussion. However, the authors seem to have struggled, for instance, to provide strong hypotheses to explain why the NY SAFE Act was associated with a significant drop in firearms-related homicides but not suicide rates. Here I elaborate on both contributions.

IMPROVING THE INTERNAL VALIDITY OF EVALUATION STUDIES

Laws such as the NY SAFE Act have been introduced not only in the United States but also in Canada, Australia, and New Zealand.[1] Several systematic reviews have been conducted to estimate the impact of multicomponent laws.[1–4] These reviews reached different conclusions about the potential of multicomponent laws to prevent firearm-related deaths. However, they all concluded that high-quality research was needed. Although some evaluation studies reported that the simultaneous implementation of laws targeting multiple elements of firearm regulations reduced firearm-related deaths in certain countries, Santaella et al. mentioned that "challenges in ecological design and the execution of studies [limit] the confidence in study findings and the conclusions that can be derived from them."[1(p152)] Important threats to internal validity have been identified in several evaluations of gun control laws.[1,2,4]

The evaluation of the NY SAFE Act was based on an innovative quasi-experimental approach to obtaining results with strong internal validity. Karaye et al. were among the first researchers to use the synthetic control method to construct a counterfactual that closely resembles the "treatment" state. The authors used data from a pool of donors—potential control states—and from the pretreatment period to predict what would have happened without the introduction of the NY SAFE Act in 2013. They were able to build a synthetic control region that was similar to the actual state of New York in terms of pretreatment sociodemographic characteristics and mortality rates. Their findings provide strong evidence about the preventive impact of the NY SAFE Act on firearm-related homicides, especially given that no substitution effect was detected. Their study paves the way for future evaluations of gun control laws based on strong quasi-experimental designs.

PREVENTIVE MECHANISMS TRIGGERED BY GUN CONTROL LAWS

Karaye et al.'s discussion shows that additional research needs to be conducted to obtain a comprehensive understanding of the impact of the NY

SAFE Act and other similar laws. As suggested by the authors, future studies could evaluate the effect of the act on nonfatal firearm-related injuries and consider individual data. In addition to such suggestions, there is an urgent need for studies that would provide an understanding of the preventive mechanisms that were associated with the decline in firearm-related homicide rates.

There is, at best, scarce knowledge on the cumulative effects of gun control laws, on how provisions are enforced by competent authorities, and on how components of gun control laws interact. To claim that a "treatment" is associated with an outcome, one must not only observe a significant relationship but also be able to provide a credible explanation. This is a basic rule of causal inference. The explanations provided by the authors in interpreting the impact of the NY SAFE Act on suicides and homicides could benefit from new evidence. At least two claims can be challenged on the basis of actual scientific evidence.

First, the authors stressed that the provisions prohibiting some assault weapons and large-capacity magazines could partially explain the observed decrease in firearm-related homicides. These weapons can contribute to mass shootings. The authors' claims are questionable. On one hand, the effect of the NY SAFE Act on mass shooting incidents or other indicators (e.g., the number of victims per incident) was not assessed. On the other hand, despite some encouraging findings about the preventive effects of banning large-capacity magazines,[5] systematic reviews are not in agreement about the impact of gun and ammunition bans. Two systematic reviews were unable to reach conclusions about the impact of such measures because evaluation studies lacked internal validity.[1,2] One review indicated that these measures are ineffective[6] and another that they are in fact effective.[7] Updating these systematic reviews with recent evaluation studies could lead to different conclusions about the impact on gun violence of banning large-capacity ammunition magazines and semiautomatic weapons.

Second, conversely to the homicide rate, suicides did not decline after the introduction of the NY SAFE Act. According to the authors, the effects on suicides could be delayed as suicide prevention efforts involve comprehensive strategies, including improved access to mental health services, community support, and efforts to reduce the stigma associated with mental health issues. This claim is delicate and debatable in it applies to homicide as well. The authors' message may also be misinterpreted: prevention of homicide goes beyond mere gun control strategies.

Several authors have stressed that prevention of firearm-related homicides needs to be multifaceted and based on a public health approach.[8] Accordingly, gun control strategies represent one approach among others. Other prevention measures have proven effective, including law enforcement strategies such as programs based on the focused-deterrence approach,[9] prevention projects offered to at-risk youths or youths in high-risk communities,[10] education campaigns promoting safe storage conditions,[11] and place-based measures such as greening efforts.[12] States should consider not only multicomponent laws in their strategy to reduce gun violence but also programs supporting primary, secondary, and tertiary prevention efforts directed at various targets (at-risk youths, blighted vacant lands, potential victims, guns). Considering the polarization of the gun control debate in the United States, researchers and experts need to promote a holistic and intersectoral approach to the prevention of firearm-related violence.[8]

In conclusion, the Karaye et al. evaluation study provides convincing results regarding the potential of multicomponent gun control laws. Their discussion highlights that there is an urgent need for additional research to build a stronger body of evidence about these laws. More precisely, their discussion shows that additional studies are needed to pinpoint the preventive mechanisms responsible for the decline in firearm-related homicide rates. Similarly, knowledge is scarce about the cumulative effects of gun control laws and other violence reduction measures. Additional knowledge on this latest issue would help further support a multifaceted approach to the prevention of gun violence. AJPH

CORRESPONDENCE

Correspondence should be sent to Etienne Blais, PhD, 3150 rue Jean-Brillant, Room C4117, Montreal, Quebec, Canada, H3T 1N8 (e-mail: etienne.blais@umontreal.ca). Reprints can be ordered at http://www.ajph.org by clicking the "Reprints" link.

PUBLICATION INFORMATION

Full Citation: Blais E. Supporting multicomponent gun control laws: a need for valid and comprehensive research. *Am J Public Health*. 2023;113(12):1238–1240.

Acceptance Date: August 19, 2023.

DOI: https://doi.org/10.2105/AJPH.2023.307431

CONFLICTS OF INTEREST

The author declares no conflicts of interest.

REFERENCES

1. Santaella-Tenorio J, Cerdá M, Villaveces A, Galea S. What do we know about the association between firearm legislation and firearm-related injuries? *Epidemiol Rev*. 2016;38(1):140–157. https://doi.org/10.1093/epirev/mxv012
2. Hahn RA, Bilukha O, Crosby A, et al. Firearms laws and the reduction of violence: a systematic

review. *Am J Prev Med.* 2005;28(2):40–71. https://doi.org/10.1016/j.amepre.2004.10.005

3. McPhedran S. A systematic review of quantitative evidence about the impacts of Australian legislative reform on firearm homicide. Available at: https://www.sciencedirect.com/science/article/abs/pii/S1359178916300258. Accessed June 20, 2023.
4. Bennett N, Karkada M, Erdogan M, Green RS. The effect of legislation on firearm-related deaths in Canada: a systematic review. *CMAJ Open.* 2022;10(2):E500–E507. https://doi.org/10.9778/cmajo.20210192
5. Siegel M, Goder-Reiser M, Duwe G, Rocque M, Fox JA, Fridel EE. The relation between state gun laws and the incidence and severity of mass public shootings in the United States, 1976–2018. *Law Hum Behav.* 2020;44(5):347–360. https://doi.org/10.1037/lhb0000378
6. Lee LK, Fleegler EW, Farrell C, et al. Firearm laws and firearm homicides: a systematic review. *JAMA Intern Med.* 2017;177(1):106–119. https://doi.org/10.1001/jamainternmed.2016.7051
7. Makarios MD, Pratt TC. The effectiveness of policies and programs that attempt to reduce firearm violence: a meta-analysis. *Crime Delinq.* 2012;58(2):222–244. https://doi.org/10.1177/0011128708321321
8. Cook PJ. Expanding the public health approach to gun violence prevention. *Ann Intern Med.* 2018;169(10):723–724. https://doi.org/10.7326/M18-2846
9. Braga AA, Cook PJ. *Policing Gun Violence: Strategic Reforms for Controlling Our Most Pressing Crime Problem.* New York, NY: Oxford University Press; 2023.
10. Petrosino A, Campie P, Pace J, et al. Cross-sector, multi-agency interventions to address urban youth firearms violence: a rapid evidence assessment. *Aggress Violent Behav.* 2015;22:87–96. https://doi.org/10.1016/j.avb.2015.04.001
11. Rowhani-Rahbar A, Simonetti JA, Rivara FP. Effectiveness of interventions to promote safe firearm storage. *Epidemiol Rev.* 2016;38(1):111–124. https://doi.org/10.1093/epirev/mxv006
12. Moyer R, MacDonald JM, Ridgeway G, Branas CC. Effect of remediating blighted vacant land on shootings: a citywide cluster randomized trial. *Am J Public Health.* 2019;109(1):140–144. https://doi.org/10.2105/AJPH.2018.304752

From *Roe* to *Dobbs*: The Critical Role of Medical Housing for Individuals Seeking Abortion Care

Jennifer A. Owens, ScD, MS, Flavius R. W. Lilly, PhD, MA, MPH, Amanda Allen, JD, Marisa Falcon, and Roger J. Ward, EdD, JD, MSL, MPA

ABOUT THE AUTHORS

Jennifer A. Owens, Flavius R. W. Lilly, and Roger J. Ward are with the University of Maryland Graduate School at the University of Maryland, Baltimore. Amanda Allen is with The Lawyering Project in Brooklyn, NY. Marisa Falcon is with Apiary for Practical Support in New York, NY.

The year 2022 marked a pivotal shift in abortion rights in the United States. In its ruling on *Dobbs v Jackson Women's Health Organization*, the Supreme Court overturned the constitutional guarantee to abortion established in *Roe v Wade*.[1] In the wake of that decision, the need for temporary medical housing has surged, as individuals are now compelled to journey considerable distances to "access states" where abortion remains legal. These individuals often need overnight accommodations to access abortion care.

Traveling for abortion care is not a new phenomenon, but, since *Dobbs*, additional tens of thousands of Americans have been forced to leave their home state to obtain abortion care.[2,3] Veritably, individuals forced to travel for abortion care are faced with unique barriers to health care access, and the distances individuals are traveling are significant. In Texas, for example, progressively more restrictive bans have impacted the average forced travel distance to the nearest abortion clinic, and this is further compounded because of neighboring states restricting abortion access. Before the Supreme Court ruling, Texans seeking abortion care traveled an average of 12 miles for care. Now, as Texas and other states have instituted abortion bans, individuals need to reach facilities in often far-reaching access states, increasing the average distance to 498.78 miles and average travel time to more than seven hours (https://bit.ly/46yvfbx).[4]

Because of this, the need to secure housing for abortion care has amplified considerably. Procedures previously within a few hours' drive may now require overnight stays or even extend over multiple days in unfamiliar cities.[5] This often involves securing a hotel or comparable accommodations, a process fraught with its own logistical and financial challenges, such as identity requirements, credit card usage, and age restrictions. Furthermore, some clinics require their patients to remain nearby during their care, which adds additional logistical complexity. This can pose an overwhelming burden for many individuals, highlighting housing support as an essential social and practical need.

ABORTION EXCEPTIONALISM TO HEALTH EQUITY

Abortion, despite being an essential component of evidence-based health care, is uniquely subjected to distinct legal, political, and social scrutiny because of abortion exceptionalism—the treatment of abortion as a unique and stigmatized issue setting it apart from other forms of health care.[6] This different treatment, manifesting since the *Roe* ruling, and further exacerbated after *Dobbs*, results in restrictive policies and limited access to abortion services even in states where it remains legal.[7] By framing abortion as a morally charged controversy instead of a routine medical intervention, it obstructs the integration of abortion care into mainstream health care systems and social safety nets such as medical housing, exacerbating health disparities and perpetuating social inequalities.[6]

To address these challenges and inequities, it is crucial for clinicians, health care leaders, and abortion care advocates to join forces with policymakers to dismantle barriers confronting individuals who must travel for abortion care. However, this requires a critical and strategic shift in perspective—from the narrative of abortion exceptionalism to the lens of health equity. This perspective recognizes health equity as an ethical and human rights principle that inspires efforts to eliminate health disparities adversely affecting marginalized or excluded groups.[8] This shift would allow for a systematic approach to measure and document the negative consequences of abortion exceptionalism, such as social exclusion, marginalization, decriminalization, and disadvantage.

The journey to access abortion care presents other significant challenges,

AJPH December 2023, Vol 113, No. 12

marked by aggressive protestors, safety risks, and an alarming increase in harassment and violence at clinics, as reported by the National Abortion Federation in 2021.[9] Coupled with geographical and environmental factors, like some clinics' locations being distant from metropolitan areas or hospitals where medical housing may exist, these challenges directly affect the viability of medical housing for abortion seekers. For instance, after *Dobbs*, more clinics have opened in smaller communities that border ban states ranging from Moorhead, Minnesota, to Carbondale, Illinois, to Cumberland, Maryland.[10–12] These challenges simultaneously underscore the need for and difficulty in implementing medical housing for abortion patients.

MEDICAL HOUSING FOR ABORTION IN PRACTICE

Medical housing has long been a recognized social need for many other health diagnoses, and numerous organizations address this need for specific health conditions and populations. Examples include the American Cancer Society, providing housing for cancer patients traveling for care, and the Ronald McDonald House Charities, which offers accommodations for children and their families during medical treatment. However, abortion care is different in some key ways from other forms of medical care for which medical housing is already established. For example, 95% of abortions in the United States are performed in abortion clinics as opposed to hospitals,[13] in contrast with other specialized medical care such as cancer care. In further contrast, individuals traveling for abortion care typically require accommodation for one to three days, wherein prolonged housing stays may be necessary for other health conditions. Furthermore, housing for abortion care is often arranged by grassroots practical support organizations (PSOs), which offer housing support as part of an array of assistance to patients, encompassing transportation, lodging, financial backing, childcare, emotional support, and advocacy. The primary objective of PSOs is to diminish logistical and financial obstacles that could impede individuals from obtaining abortion care.

Currently, more than 60 organizations provide practical support for abortion care nationwide (https://bit.ly/46NhVjj). Their scope ranges from grassroots organizations, such as the Haven Coalition in New York City, comprising volunteer housing hosts, to more comprehensive organizations like the Midwest Access Coalition and Brigid Alliance. To manage their clients' unique circumstances, PSOs prioritize their interest and safety, often preferring hotels over volunteer housing for privacy and anonymity. To streamline the process and preserve client confidentiality, PSOs often book lodging on behalf of their clients. To further protect the privacy of clients, PSOs often use work-arounds such as booking under the names of companions or using programs like SafeStays, which is a service to anonymously book hotels for abuse survivors and now is frequently used for abortion care. This crucial support, in conjunction with coordinating other needs such as travel, food, and childcare, ensures that individuals can access their appointments with a secure place to stay.

There has been a call for clinicians and health care leaders to collaborate with advocates and policymakers to reduce barriers for individuals traveling for abortion and advocate proactive policies to expand care, as well as financially support abortion funds and practical support organizations.[14] To better support adequate and sustainable medical housing for abortion seekers, we recommend the following:

Policy and Systems

- Incorporate a housing in health strategy that recognizes medical housing as a critical component of public health.
- Develop policy frameworks that protect and promote access to medical housing for individuals seeking abortion care.
- Audit current housing resources and conduct needs assessments, so health care and policy leaders understand the medical housing ecosystems in their area and which resources are available to support individuals traveling for abortion care.

Human-Centeredness

- Center the needs of those traveling for abortion care, keeping in mind each person's needs are different and many may prefer an anonymous and private setting as opposed to a group setting model used by other models of medical housing.
- Ensure continuity of care by ensuring coordinated postprocedure care and support, including housing needs, especially those who have traveled far from home.
- Conduct training programs for health care staff on the specific needs and concerns of individuals traveling for abortion care.

Partnership and Collaboration

- Encourage leaders who support medical housing for other diagnoses to partner with PSOs. Health care leaders in all states should form regional alliances and invite medical housing experts to the table to collaborate on ways to reduce travel burdens for those seeking abortion care.
- Fund organizations that provide temporary housing for individuals traveling for abortion care.

Given the current crisis in abortion access, it is essential to meet the housing needs of those traveling for abortion care while simultaneously acknowledging the unique factors introduced by abortion exceptionalism and the politicized environment surrounding abortion rights. Advocates need to work toward creating more comprehensive and supportive policies that address the holistic needs of people seeking abortion services. AJPH

CORRESPONDENCE

Correspondence should be sent to Jennifer A. Owens, ScD, MS, University of Maryland, Baltimore, Graduate School, 620 W Lexington St, Suite 102, Baltimore, MD 21210 (e-mail: jowens@umaryland.edu). Reprints can be ordered at https://ajph.org by clicking the "Reprints" link.

PUBLICATION INFORMATION

Full Citation: Owens JA, Lilly Flavius R. W., Allen A, Falcon M, Ward RJ. From *Roe* to *Dobbs*: the critical role of medical housing for individuals seeking abortion care. *Am J Public Health*. 2023;113(12):1241–1243.

Acceptance Date: September 16, 2023.

DOI: https://doi.org/10.2105/AJPH.2023.307464

CONTRIBUTORS

J. A. Owens, F. R. W. Lilly, A. Allen, M. Falcon, and R. J. Ward collectively contributed to this opinion editorial. J. A. Owens initiated and conceptualized the project. J. A. Owens actively sought out and collaborated with experts in abortion care to ensure a comprehensive and multidisciplinary approach to the issue. F. R. W. Lilly, A. Allen, M. Falcon, and R. J. Ward each played a crucial role in advancing our understanding of the important public health issues addressed in this article and further participated in manuscript development and revision. We deliberately cultivated a group with different perspectives and experiences in research and in practice.

CONFLICTS OF INTEREST

J. A. Owens volunteers her time on the evenings and weekends leading a medical housing support organization called Hosts for Humanity, located in Baltimore, Maryland.

REFERENCES

1. Palacio H. Over the precipice into a post-*Roe* world—a look at abortion rights and access in the United States. *Am J Public Health*. 2022;112(9):1273–1275. https://doi.org/10.2105/AJPH.2022.307016
2. Koerth M, Thomson-DeVeaux A. Over 66,000 people couldn't get an abortion in their home state after Dobbs. FiveThirtyEight. April 11, 2023. Available at: https://fivethirtyeight.com/features/post-dobbs-abortion-access-66000. Accessed June 1, 2023.
3. Smith MH, Muzyczka Z, Chakraborty P, Johns-Wolfe E, Higgins J, Bessett D, Norris AH. Abortion travel within the United States: an observational study of cross-state movement to obtain abortion care in 2017. *Lancet Reg Health Am*. 2022;10:100214. https://doi.org/10.1016/j.lana.2022.100214.
4. Bearak J, Jones RK, Nash E, Donovan MK. COVID-19 abortion bans would greatly increase driving distances for those seeking care. New York, NY: The Guttmacher Institute; 2020.
5. Kimport K. Reducing the burdens of forced abortion travel: referrals, financial and emotional support, and opportunities for positive experiences in traveling for third-trimester abortion care. *Soc Sci Med*. 2022;293:114667. https://doi.org/10.1016/j.socscimed.2021.114667
6. Donley G. Medication abortion exceptionalism. *Cornell Law Rev*. 2021;107(3):627–704. Available at: https://live-cornell-law-review.pantheonsite.io/wp-content/uploads/2022/06/Donley-final.pdf. Accessed October 23, 2023.
7. Fox D, Cole E. The Supreme Court's abortion exceptionalism—judicial deference, medical science, and mifepristone access. *N Engl J Med*. 2021;384(24):e94. https://doi.org/10.1056/NEJMp2104461
8. Braveman P, Arkin E, Orleans T, Proctor D, Plough A. *What Is Health Equity? And What Difference Does a Definition Make?* Princeton, NJ: Robert Wood Johnson Foundation; 2017:3.
9. National Abortion Federation. 2021 violence and disruption statistics. 2021. Available at: https://prochoice.org/wp-content/uploads/2021_NAF_VD_Stats_Final.pdf. Accessed May 23, 2023.
10. Witt E. An abortion clinic one year later. *The New Yorker*. 2023. Available at: https://www.newyorker.com/news/us-journal/an-abortion-clinic-one-year-later. Accessed September 6, 2023.
11. Sasani A, Schaff E. When the abortion clinic came to town. *New York Times*. November 30, 2022. Available at: https://www.nytimes.com/2022/11/30/us/abortion-clinic-illinois.html. Accessed September 6, 2023.
12. Willingham L. New Maryland provider opening in post-Roe "abortion desert." *AP News*. March 27. 2023. Available at: https://apnews.com/article/maryland-abortion-clinic-west-virginia-647cbd9eccfaaa740e523a5c39208b19. Accessed September 6, 2023.
13. Jones RK, Witwer E, Jerman J. Abortion incidence and service availability in the United States, 2017. September 2019 report. Available at: https://www.guttmacher.org/report/abortion-incidence-service-availability-us-2017. Accessed January 25, 2023.
14. Grossman D, Perritt J, Grady D. The impending crisis of access to safe abortion care in the US. *JAMA Intern Med*. 2022;182(8):793–795. https://doi.org/10.1001/jamainternmed.2022.2893

Overcoming Barriers to Training the Next Generation of Public Health Professionals

Saara Z. Nasruddin, PharmD, MS, Tess Johnson, MS, Melissa Presley, MPH, Breanna Wade, MS, Quest Whalen, MS, Elizabeth Gordineer, BS, Caroline Compretta, PhD, Erin Dehon, PhD, Allison Ford-Wade, PhD, Murrell Godfrey, PhD, and Marie Barnard, PhD

ABOUT THE AUTHORS

Saara Z. Nasruddin, Tess Johnson, and Marie Barnard are with the Department of Pharmacy Administration, School of Pharmacy, University of Mississippi, University. Melissa Presley and Allison Ford-Wade are with the Department of Health, Exercise Science, and Recreation Management, School of Applied Sciences, University of Mississippi. Breanna Wade and Caroline Compretta are with the Department of Population Health Science, John D. Bower School of Population Health, University of Mississippi Medical Center, Jackson. Quest Whalen is with the Department of Data Science, John D. Bower School of Population Health, University of Mississippi Medical Center. Elizabeth Gordineer is with the Department of Neurosurgery, School of Medicine, University of Mississippi Medical Center. Erin Dehon is with the Department of Emergency Medicine, School of Medicine, University of Mississippi Medical Center. Murrell Godfrey is with the Department of Chemistry and Biochemistry, College of Liberal Arts, University of Mississippi.

AJPH December 2023, Vol 113, No. 12

Mississippi consistently ranks as one of the least healthy states in the United States (https://bit.ly/4647kAs). In 2017, Mississippi had the highest death rate in the nation from heart and kidney disease, and the second highest from stroke, diabetes, cancer, influenza or pneumonia, and septicemia (https://bit.ly/3LIu5BR). According to the America's Health Rankings 2022 annual report, approximately 12.4% of Mississippians have cardiovascular disease and 15.2% have diabetes, ranking Mississippi at 48th in the nation on both measures. Compared with the rest of the nation, Mississippians are the most likely to be born at a low birth weight (Mississippi: 11.8%; United States: 8.2% of infants weighing less than 2500 grams at birth; https://bit.ly/48sx9fh) and die a premature death (Mississippi: 13 781 years; United States: 8659 years of potential life lost before age 75 per 100 000 population annually; https://bit.ly/3tcXPR1). In addition, Mississippi had one of the highest rates of obesity, with 39.1% of the state categorized as obese.[1] From health behaviors, like smoking and physical activity, to lack of health care access, Mississippians are burdened with excess disease, much of which is associated with factors that are preventable and modifiable. These poor health indicators are not confined to Mississippi's adults.

HEALTH STATUS AND BEHAVIORS OF MISSISSIPPI YOUTHS

Undeniably, when compared with youths in other states, Mississippi youths engage in and experience significantly riskier health behaviors. Data from the Centers for Disease Control and Prevention's 2019 Youth Risk Behavior Survey show that, compared with youths in the rest of the country, Mississippi youths report statistically significant higher levels of rarely or never wearing seatbelts (Mississippi: 9.9%; United States: 6.5%); sexual activity before age 13 years (Mississippi: 5.4%; United States: 3.0%); sexually risky behaviors, such as no condom use in last sexual encounter (Mississippi: 51.6%; United States: 45.7%); and attempted suicide (Mississippi: 12.7%; United States: 8.9%).[2] In addition, Mississippi youths have statistically significant higher levels of reporting not eating fruit (Mississippi: 10.7%; United States: 6.3%) or vegetables (Mississippi: 16.0%; United States: 7.9%) in the past week, not participating in 60 minutes of physical activity on any day in the past week (Mississippi: 20.4%; United States: 17.0%), and drinking soda one or more times per day (Mississippi: 24.7%; United States: 15.1%).[2]

Despite efforts by state and community agencies to promote healthy behaviors through educational and interventional programs over the past 20 years, there has been little evidence that any of these initiatives have been effective at reducing risky health behaviors among Mississippi's youths. Trend data show that rates of child and adolescent obesity, suicidal behaviors, unhealthy eating, physical inactivity, sex without a condom, and carrying a weapon have increased from 2003 to 2019.[2] These unhealthy behaviors contribute to the leading causes of excess morbidity and mortality among Mississippi's youths—obesity, diabetes, asthma, sexually transmitted infections, motor vehicle accidents, homicide, and suicide.[3,4]

BARRIERS TO STEM CAREERS FOR MISSISSIPPIANS

Systemic inequities in access to health care and quality educational opportunity for the youth of Mississippi are powerful forces that disengage students from entering pathways toward science, technology, engineering, and mathematics (STEM) careers. On nearly all indicators related to STEM preparedness, Mississippi consistently ranks as the worst or nearly the worst in the United States. Only 20% of Mississippi eighth graders demonstrated science proficiency.[5] In 2022, only 42.9% of Mississippi students met the national standard for college and career readiness.[6] This impacts the STEM pipeline. In 2021, the rate of Bachelor's degrees in science and engineering conferred was only 17.96 per 1000 individuals aged 18 to 24 years compared with the national rate of 25.51 per 1000.[5]

Even more disheartening, the average undergraduate tuition at a public four-year institution was 45.9% of disposable personal income, one of the highest rates in the nation.[5] For most Mississippi students, unless they are aware of and have the ability to seek out financial resources, the STEM pathway ends before even entering college. Of STEM degrees awarded from the state's public institutions of higher learning in 2022, 27.8% were earned by Black students, although approximately 38% of the state's population is Black.[7,8] In 2020, Mississippi had the lowest rates of individuals in STEM occupations as a percentage of all occupations in the nation (Mississippi: 2.69%; United States: 5.26%).[5] Perhaps most worrisome for the biomedical workforce, in 2020, Mississippi had far fewer individuals in the life (0.28%) and social sciences (0.14%) fields than in other STEM fields.[5] These data indicate there is a need to broaden the conversation from STEM in general and warrants focus on public health, including the life and social and behavioral sciences.

OPPORTUNITIES TO ENGAGE STUDENTS IN PUBLIC HEALTH

Project SCORE (Student Centered Outcomes Research Experience) is a National Institutes of Health Science Education Partnership Award project that engages students from groups underrepresented in STEM career trajectories through a youth participatory action research approach. Guided by this approach, Project SCORE leverages a near-peer mentor model to engage and support underrepresented students in an exploration of the field of public health. Project SCORE brings together underrepresented high school and graduate health sciences students within two Mississippi communities (Oxford and Jackson) that experience health disparities. Each of these sites participates in a year-long weekly afterschool program to develop health behavior research questions, provide training in research methods, and facilitate the development of student-conducted research projects mentored by near-peer graduate health sciences students and faculty. A student-centered research agenda is being developed to support future research initiatives. This project seeks to increase awareness of and interest in public health, science engagement, and STEM careers, as well as increase matriculation into higher-education STEM programs to enhance and diversify the future biomedical workforce.

However, this program, which aims to introduce high school students to public health and social determinants of health (SDOH), was affected by these very issues in implementation. This article describes the SDOH that affected the implementation of Project SCORE and the adaptations made in response to these implementation challenges.

A NEED FOR EMERGENCY PREPAREDNESS AND BROADBAND ACCESS

COVID-19 impacted not only formal education and learning but also informal afterschool learning opportunities, like Project SCORE, which provides students with individualized attention and supplemental knowledge and experiences. In August 2021, when Project SCORE initially aimed to start, the Delta wave of COVID-19 hit Mississippi.[9] On August 12, 2021, the Mississippi State Department of Health released a statement on Twitter: "Today the state has surpassed all previous highs in Mississippians hospitalized for COVID-19. Hospitals are operating at emergency capacity to cope with the incoming flood of COVID-19 patients."[10] While the Mississippi governor extended the public health emergency for another 30 days, no mask mandates nor any lockdown regulations were included in the declaration.[11] The Mississippi Board of Education allowed for hybrid schooling, but each county and district chose how to implement this rule.

While hybrid and virtual education options were needed, Internet access in communities such as Jackson,

Mississippi, were poor for many residents. Approximately 20% of Mississippians do not have access to broadband Internet, the highest without broadband access compared with Mississippi's neighboring states of Alabama (12.4%), Louisiana (11.6%), Arkansas (19%), and Tennessee (6.3%).[12] When schools transitioned to virtual learning, informal education, such as afterschool activities, halted. Project SCORE was unable to operate because the needed COVID-19 restrictions prevented team members from physically interacting with the community to recruit participants. Informal learning opportunities are significant to adolescent development, helping adolescents develop social and emotional learning.[13] Social and emotional competencies are important in adolescent development of responsibility, healthy relationships with others, and achieving personal goals.[13] Afterschool activities also provide adolescents with additional academic support, expose them to opportunities they may not have found on their own, and help them to see themselves in roles they may not have envisioned for themselves.[13]

Because of safety concerns, the Project SCORE team halted programing for fall 2021. The team continued to monitor the COVID-19 outbreak and worked with community leaders to reset a goal to implement programming in spring 2022. While the Project SCORE team worked during fall 2021 to aim for a spring 2022 start to the program, the shift to virtual communication because of the COVID-19 pandemic came with challenges of coordinating with community leaders. Because community leaders manage the day-to-day operations of the community center in person, attempting to reach community leaders by e-mail, the method of communication most used by academics, posed a challenge. In-person interactions with community leaders were most effective in planning strategies to implement programming. Community leaders can disseminate information about programming with community members and effectively recruit participants into the program by word of mouth. However, because of the need to prioritize safety during this time, SCORE team members delayed in-person interactions until COVID-19 cases in the community were low.

After much planning and deliberation, Project SCORE was able to start programming in spring 2022. With the aim of making public health tangible and actionable, on the first day of Project SCORE, team members and students built Corsi–Rosenthal boxes, homemade air filters shown to reduce exposure to COVID-19 transmission.[14] Team members taught students how the Corsi–Rosenthal box works to clean the air and the importance of protective measures such as masking and air filters to reduce virus transmission during the COVID-19 pandemic.

CLIMATE CHANGE AND INCONSISTENT ENGAGEMENT

In addition to navigating the uncertainty of the pandemic, an unexpected challenge that arose during this time was inclement weather. There were 76 tornado warnings within five weeks in the state, more warnings than were issued by any other National Weather Service office in the country.[15,16]

Implementing the first sessions of Project SCORE, in which team members were in the vital stage of building relationships with the high school participants and developing trust with the community, was challenging. Sessions were inconsistent because of storm and tornado warnings that were issued each week from March 22, 2022, through April 17, 2022.[15] Some of these warnings led to school or afterschool closings, which canceled and delayed sessions with the students.[15] Because of the inconsistency of sessions with the students, lessons were unable to build upon each other each week, which hindered engagement. These challenges resulted in the Project SCORE team revising lessons to account for reviewing previous material and incorporated games and physical activity into lessons to improve engagement and foster community with the students.

WATER SYSTEM INFRASTRUCTURE CRISIS EFFECTS FOR STUDENTS

Jackson reached national headlines in August 2022 when flood waters overwhelmed the city's water treatment system, cutting off water pressure and leaving 150 000 Jackson residents without access to safe drinking water for weeks.[17,18] Since 2018, the city has been in violation of safe drinking water standards.[19] Jackson residents regularly experience sewer line breaks, boil water notices, and exposure to toxic bacteria in their water.[19] For decades, it has been known that the original water infrastructure, laid out more than a century ago, needed to be replaced.[19,20] However, the cost for improvements is about $1 billion, and infrastructure improvements have been postponed because of increased poverty associated with reduced revenue streams in the city.[19] In addition, the city struggles to hire and retain water and sewer operators and staff, which contributes to the deterioration of the water quality, another indication of the need to build the STEM pipeline in Mississippi.[19]

Because of the water crisis, Jackson public schools were unable to operate facilities, and students were switched back to virtual learning in August 2023.[21] Project SCORE's Jackson community partner was unable to offer afterschool programming for weeks. During this time, when the Oxford team launched programming, the Jackson team had to allocate their time to figure out how to consistently obtain clean water for the participants. The Jackson team had no choice but to halt afterschool programming until the community partner was able to safely reopen the building and services. The Oxford team provided the Jackson team with an excess supply of bottled water, which was handed out to the Jackson SCORE students each session.

CONCLUSION

The implementation of an afterschool program aimed at enhancing the STEM pipeline and addressing health inequities in Mississippi was affected by some of the very SDOH it aimed to mitigate. Programs in which the immediate results may not be actualized but are nevertheless needed to address disparities in the long term must adapt and overcome the same barriers that caused the poor outcomes. In Mississippi, these SDOH included broadband Internet access, water infrastructure, climate change, and public health, which need to be addressed on different levels—from government and policy to individual attitudes. Projects that aim to highlight these issues to adolescents, who have had to adapt to these conditions and may not fully recognize the severity of these SDOH, are needed. These projects require resiliency and support to achieve the long-term results that will make a difference in health inequities. AJPH

CORRESPONDENCE

Correspondence should be sent to Saara Z. Nasruddin, 207 Hathorn Rd, Oxford, MS 38655 (e-mail: snasrudd@go.olemiss.edu). Reprints can be ordered at https://ajph.org by clicking the "Reprints" link.

PUBLICATION INFORMATION

Full Citation: Nasruddin SZ, Johnson T, Presley M, et al. Overcoming barriers to training the next generation of public health professionals. *Am J Public Health*. 2023;113(12):1244–1248.

Acceptance Date: August 8, 2023.

DOI: https://doi.org/10.2105/AJPH.2023.307412

CONTRIBUTORS

S. Z. Nasruddin and M. Barnard originated the commentary concept and drafted the article. T. Johnson, M. Presley, B. Wade, Q. Whalen, E. Gordineer, C. Compretta, E. Dehon, A. Ford-Wade, and M. Godfrey participated in data collection, analysis, and article review.

ACKNOWLEDGMENTS

This project is funded by a Science Education Partnership Award from the National Institute of General Medical Sciences at the National Institutes of Health.

CONFLICTS OF INTEREST

The authors have no conflicts of interest to disclose.

REFERENCES

1. America's Health Rankings. Explore health measures in Mississippi. 2021 Annual Report. Available at: https://www.americashealthrankings.org/explore/annual/state/MS. Accessed September 15, 2022.
2. Mississippi State Department of Health Bureau of Vital Statistics. Youth Risk Behavior Survey 2019. Available at: https://msdh.ms.gov/msdhsite/index.cfm/31,19694,302,pdf/2019_Youth_Risk_behavior_report.pdf. Accessed May 15, 2023.
3. Walker V. Mississippi Child Death Review Panel 2022 Annual Report. Available at: https://msdh.ms.gov/msdhsite/index.cfm/31,18967,392,pdf/2022_CDR_Report_Draft_revised.pdf. Accessed May 15, 2023.
4. Children's Safety Network Economics and Data Analysis Resource Center. Children's Safety Network state fact sheets—Mississippi. Calverton, MD: Pacific Institute for Research and Evaluation; 2106.
5. National Science Foundation. Science and engineering state indicators—Mississippi. Available at: https://ncses.nsf.gov/indicators/states/state/mississippi. Accessed May 15, 2023.
6. Mississippi Department of Education. Mississippi Succeeds Report Card. Available at: https://msrc.mdek12.org. Accessed May 15, 2023.
7. Rankins A. Fast facts 2021–2022. Mississippi State Institutions of Higher Learning. Available at: https://files.eric.ed.gov/fulltext/ED617849.pdf. Accessed May 15, 2023.
8. World Population Review. Mississippi population 2023. Available at: https://worldpopulationreview.com/states/mississippi-population. Accessed May 15, 2023.
9. Delta Covid 'tsunami' hits Mississippi; Florida only has 'so many beds.' *Kaiser Health News*. August 6, 2021. Available at: https://khn.org/morning-breakout/delta-covid-tsunami-hits-mississippi-florida-only-has-so-many-beds. Accessed February 22, 2023.
10. @msdh. Today the state has surpassed all previous highs in Mississippians hospitalized for COVID-19. Hospitals are operating at emergency capacity to cope with the incoming flood of COVID-19 patients. Of the nearly 1,500 now in a hospital for COVID-19, more than 1,300 are unvaccinated. Twitter. August 12, 2021. Available at: https://twitter.com/msdh/status/1425896724564959239. Accessed February 22, 2023.
11. Sanderlin LO. Governor extends emergency declaration amid newest COVID-19 surge to ensure federal help. *Clarion Ledger*. Available at: https://www.clarionledger.com/story/news/2021/08/12/reeves-extend-emergency-orders-covid-19-ravages/8110672002. Accessed March 7, 2023.
12. Mississippi State University Extension Service. The state of broadband access in Mississippi. Available at: http://extension.msstate.edu/publications/the-state-broadband-access-mississippi. Accessed May 17, 2023.
13. Youth.gov. Benefits for youth, families, and communities. Available at: https://youth.gov/youth-topics/afterschool-programs/benefits-youth-families-and-communities. Accessed April 8, 2023.
14. Dodson RE, Manz KE, Burks SR, et al. Does using Corsi–Rosenthal boxes to mitigate COVID-19 transmission also reduce indoor air concentrations of PFAS and phthalates? *Environ Sci Technol*. 2023;57(1):415–427. https://doi.org/10.1021/acs.est.2c05169
15. Nasruddin S, Presley M, Wahlen Q, et al. Implementing health sciences after-school programming for Mississippi high school students: the impact of social determinants of health. University of Mississippi, Annual Poster Session 2022. October 11, 2022. Available at: https://egrove.olemiss.edu/pharm_annual_posters_2022/14. Accessed April 15, 2023.

16. Gray J. Central Mississippi faced 76 tornadoes in just 35 days this spring. *CNN*. April 25, 2022. Available at: https://www.cnn.com/2022/04/25/weather/weather-news-record-tornadoes-wxn/index.html. Accessed October 6, 2022.
17. De La Garza A. Jackson's water crisis is a climate justice wake-up call. *Time*. September 15, 2022. Available at: https://time.com/6213616/jackson-water-crisis-environmental-justice-mississippi. Accessed October 6, 2022.
18. Engle J. Lesson plan: the Mississippi water crisis and what it means for the rest of the nation. *New York Times*. September 16, 2022. Available at: https://www.nytimes.com/2022/09/16/learning/lesson-plans/lesson-plan-the-mississippi-water-crisis-and-what-it-means-for-the-rest-of-the-nation.html. Accessed October 6, 2022.
19. Le Coz E, Connolly D, Hitson H, Mealins E. Jackson water crisis flows from century of poverty, neglect and racism. *Mississippi Today*. November 7, 2022. Available at: https://mississippitoday.org/2022/11/07/jackson-water-crisis-poverty-neglect-racism. Accessed April 4, 2023.
20. Timeline: Jackson water crisis. *Jackson Advocate*. September 22, 2022. Available at: https://jacksonadvocateonline.com/timeline-jackson-water-crisis. Accessed April 4, 2023.
21. Water crisis: Jackson closings, postponements, schools, events, athletics. *Clarion Ledger*. Available at: https://www.clarionledger.com/story/news/2022/08/31/water-crisis-jackson-ms-closings-and-postponements-schools-events-athletics/65466111007. Accessed April 8, 2023.

Typhoid Mary Was Not a Super-Spreader (and Super-Spreaders Are Not "Typhoid Marys")

Amir Teicher, PhD

ABOUT THE AUTHOR

Amir Teicher is with the Department of History, Tel Aviv University, Tel Aviv, Israel.

In discussions about super-spreaders, one figure who features prominently is "Typhoid Mary"—the Irish immigrant cook who was an asymptomatic carrier of typhoid bacilli, infected 47 people, and led to at least three deaths in early 20th-century New York State. In the past three years, references to Typhoid Mary, whose real name was Mary Mallon, as the first, most prominent, or prototypical example of a "super-spreader" are common in scientific papers, blogs, videos, podcasts, and articles in the popular press (see the Appendix, available as a supplement to the online version of this article at https://ajph.org).

Does the historical case of Mary Mallon really qualify her for such a role? The answer obviously depends on how we define super-spreaders. Contemporary applications of the term vary, but most commonly it is used to refer to individuals who instigated an "explosive outbreak" of simultaneous infections, or to the theoretical discussion of infectiousness heterogeneity in shaping the course of epidemics. Super-spreading, in the sense of actual or potential "extraordinary" infectiousness, is described as caused by (1) biological, physiological, or immunological mechanisms or (2) as grounded in social or behavioral dynamics. At first glance, Mary falls into the latter category: she was an asymptomatic carrier of *Salmonella typhi* who worked as a cook and was characterized by health officials as lacking in personal hygiene. Thus, she had all necessary qualifications to unknowingly and effectively disperse pathogens. Nonetheless, I argue that her story is hardly compatible with our contemporary understanding of super-spreading and that the tendency to associate her with the term is scientifically, historically, and morally precarious.

THE FACTS ABOUT MARY

The story of Mary Mallon is well researched and relatively familiar and will, therefore, not be reproduced here in great detail. What is important to note is that contrary to how she is sometimes portrayed, Mary did not instigate any large epidemic. When, in 1908, she first received her notorious nickname, the 22 infections traced back to her were the sum of a collection of small household outbreaks, disconnected in time and space, which occurred over the course of no less than seven years (1900–1907). Thus, she became "Typhoid Mary" before she caused any single "super-spreader event." To properly assess the singularity of these infections, it is essential to recall that at the time of Mary's arrest, typhoid fever was constantly fluctuating between an endemic state and occasional, often seasonal, epidemic outbursts. The annual toll of typhoid fever infections in the United States was in the scale of several hundreds of thousands, and in New York State alone amounted to 3500 new cases each year.[1(p49–50)] Epidemiologically, what distinguished Mary from many others was that, as a cook who relocated with each new job, her "trail of infections" could be reconstructed.

There was, however, one outbreak that Mary caused that retrospectively could be portrayed as a "super-spreader" event—but only if under the term "event" we include an occurrence lasting two months. Five years after she had been released from enforced quarantine, in 1915, an additional 25 cases and two deaths were added to her count. These occurred during a period in which Mary worked as a cook in Sloane Maternity Hospital's kitchen. The event attracted professional attention in the medical community, not so much because of its magnitude, as much as because it happened in a place where most staff were vaccinated.[2,3] Physicians and journalists perceived it as scandalous both because of the vulnerability of those affected and because it seemed to prove that Mary was untrustworthy—that she had defied her promise upon release that she would cease working as a cook.[1(p152)]

From the perspective of the early 20th century, however, the Sloane Hospital case was one among many

AJPH December 2023, Vol 113, No. 12

food-poisoning incidents—and far from the most devastating one. In 1920, for example, newspapers throughout the United States informed the American public of a mystery "poison guest" that turned a "merry luncheon party" held by wealthy women from Cleveland, Ohio, into a disaster. That guest

> haunted this fashionable society function like an angel of death, scattering the disease germs that made thirty-nine women seriously ill and ha[s] already killed two victims.[4]

Eleven years later, in 1931, American newspapers reported on

> Death at the Wedding Feast: A kindly friend of the bride's family offers to make the sandwiches and mix the chicken salad—and unconsciously she stirs into the bowl typhoid germs which lay the young bride and her sister and her aunt in their graves and stretch 24 guests on hospital beds.[5]

Mary's case pales in comparison with these horrific dramas, and, once again, differs from them in its nonsimultaneity.

There is another principal distinction between Mary's story and super-spreading: typhoid fever is not airborne, whereas the term "super-spreader" and the phenomenon of "super-spreading," are strongly related to respiratory diseases and diseases that are transmitted via the air. The first experimental evidences for heterogeneity in infectiousness, which could make particular individuals especially dangerous or efficient disease "transmitters," were obtained in the early 1960s with respect to tuberculosis aerosolization,[6] influenza spread,[7] and coxsackievirus coughs,[8] and the term "super-spreader" was itself first coined in 1972 with relation to stochastic models of influenza epidemics.[9] The term was later applied also to discuss smallpox, measles, rubella, tuberculosis, Middle East respiratory syndrome (MERS), and severe acute respiratory syndrome coronavirus (SARS-CoV)-1 and -2. Admittedly, scientists borrowed it to discuss other diseases such as gonorrhea, AIDS, and Ebola. But it was in relation to airborne transmitted diseases and the epidemiological effects of aerosolization that the phenomenon of super-spreading was scientifically recognized and the term defined and refined.

Against this background, choosing Mary Mallon as an archetypal super-spreader is indeed odd. From almost every possible perspective—public health; virology, bacteriology, and parasitology; physiology; and epidemiology, as well as sanitation and hygiene—airborne and fecal–oral transmission belong in different domains. One exception might be network theory, which, through its mathematical models, tends to view all long-tailed distributions as equivalent. Within this latter framework, super-spreaders are commonly defined as the 10% to 20% of the population who lead to 80% to 90% of infections. Such a definition, by making every fifth or tenth person a super-spreader, trivializes this concept to such an extent that it makes Mary's sensational story, once again, ill-fitted for the job.

HOW DID MARY BECOME A "SUPER-SPREADER"?

Neither a "patient zero" associated with an emerging epidemic nor a crucial link in maintaining such an epidemic, Mary was nonetheless a person who infected many others. But for medical scholars of the early 20th century, what her case stood for was very different from the current concern with super-spreaders and their role in epidemics. Mary represented another problem, which, incidentally, has been a nonissue in the COVID-19 context: that of chronic carriers, who may not be aware of ever having been ill and seed repeated small-scale outbreaks over years or even decades. The milkman or food-handler or waitress whose cousin fell ill with typhoid 10 years earlier and who has since unknowingly, slowly, but continuously infected their customers—that was the prototype revealed and embodied by Mary's figure.[10]

The novelty of the concept of asymptomatic carriers at that time brought Mary's story into focus and rendered it a case in point. Her refusal to accept her status quickly turned into a question of authority. Portraying her as a negative model-carrier served the interests of public health authorities—a moral tale with educational goals, which at the same time shifted the responsibilities for maintaining public health from governments and municipalities to individuals. For certain public health leaders, Mary's story helped to convey a new paradigm of public health, one that focused less on public sanitation and more on personal hygiene.[11] Yet, the factors that made it possible to turn her into an emblem of disease spread, while depriving her of her rights and quarantining her indefinitely, had to do more with her social attributes than anything else. Her case touched several sensitive nerves: some were related to the supposed ignorance and uncleanliness of Irish immigrants; others were to women's role in society and the various epidemiological dangers that purportedly stemmed from their dysfunctional performance as housewives and mothers. As Judith Leavitt and Priscilla Wald have shown, Mary personified the "problem" of the unmarried woman but also exemplified the consequences of the mother-in-absentia, who leaves it to a stranger to cook for her children.[1,12]

From her 1915 reapprehension onward, Mary's story acquired mythical dimensions, and her name has been repeatedly brought up in relation to a range of medical hazards. Fallaciously boosting her morbidity toll, she has occasionally been associated with a devastating 1903 outbreak of typhoid fever in Ithaca, New York, which resulted in more than 1300 cases and 82 deaths. This attribution was based on one of the accounts of George Soper, the man who identified Mary and led to her apprehension, in which he mentioned his own experiences from that 1903 outbreak.[13] In the hands of later readers, Soper's description morphed into an alleged "subsequent study" that presumably showed that

> a person by the name of Mary Mallon had been employed as a cook in the vicinity of the place where the first case [of the Ithaca outbreak] appeared, and from which contamination of the water supply occurred.[14(p724)]

This latter description, which had absolutely no known factual basis, was printed in the 1921 edition of a definitive and popular textbook, *Preventive Medicine and Hygiene* (later titled *Preventive Medicine and Public Health*), authored by Milton Rosenau, director of the Hygienic Laboratory of the US Public Health Service, who earlier gave Mary her infamous nickname.[15] The same sentences were reproduced verbatim in other academic venues, appeared in subsequent editions (up until 1956) of Rosenau's textbook, and were taken at face value in a 1967 survey on "The Scourge of Typhoid."[14,16] As said, this attribution is entirely false and based on a misunderstanding.

In parallel, Mallon's name has become a must-mention in popular descriptions of disease outbreaks. Thus, the 1920 writer on the "poison guest" called that guest a "New Typhoid Mary"[4]; the wedding feast report from 1931 also mentioned Mary and even attached her photo.[5] Such references gradually extended further. In 1939, New Jersey readers learned about "Psittacosis Polly—more menacing than Typhoid Mary." "The word may sound silly—but the danger is real . . . Typhoid Mary is dead . . . but Psittacosis Polly is very much alive and squawking."[17] Less humorous in tone, in 1948, Memphis, Tennessee, had to cope with "25 'Typhoid Marys' [who] walk streets laden with billions of germs."[18] The year 1963 saw the state of California destroying "hundreds of 'Typhoid Mary' trees," which were asymptomatic "carriers of citrus killing virus."[19] Two years later, back in New Jersey, the chairman of the Essex County Mental Health In-Patient Planning Committee warned that untreated mentally ill people could become contagious and instigate a chain of mental problems in their families and communities, in a report that received the title, "Psychotic Typhoid Mary's Help Spread Mental Disease."[20]

As these examples demonstrate, analogies to Typhoid Mary were not initiated only by sensation-seeking journalists; then as now, it was often scientists and medical professionals who raised them in the first place and who used them both in internal discussions as well as in their communications with the public. This was true, also, in relation to the discussion of "super-spreaders." In 1982, 10 years after the term "super-spreaders" began circulating among New York medical scholars, Mallon's case was raised during a "Workshop on Population Biology of Infectious Disease Agents" held in Berlin. In the context of the workshop, the term "super-spreader" stood for the idea that "certain individuals in the population may be infected, and highly infectious, for long periods of time but may exhibit no overt signs of disease."[21(p165)] In other words, in that workshop, "super-spreader" was borrowed to describe an asymptomatic chronic carrier. A report in *Nature* on that conference named "Typhoid Marys" as examples of such super-spreaders.[22]

Similar references continued, while at the same time, the meaning of "super-spreaders" shifted back to where it had begun—namely, at the acute rather than the chronic pole, and in the air-related rather than food-related domain. In the cultural sphere, Mary's story has in the meantime become a small industry, and the 1980s saw new novels and theatrical productions based loosely on her story appearing almost annually, with various moral lessons for society in the era of AIDS.[1(p202-227)] As Richard McKay and Priscilla Wald have shown, Mary's story also shaped the scientific and popular characterization of the flight attendant Gaëtan Dugas, crowned as the "Patient Zero" of the AIDS epidemic. Following the first SARS epidemic, one scholar raised Mary to the status of "patron saint of superspreaders."[23] Then in 2008, an academic book on infectious disease ecology reproduced the false accusation that Mary caused the Ithaca outbreak, defining Mary as "one of the most notorious superspreaders" and claiming that "[b]etween 1900 and 1907 she initiated twenty-eight outbreaks [should have been: cases] of typhoid fever" as well as "one outbreak in Ithaca [that] allegedly led to 1,400 people being infected."[24(p358)] Ten years ago, the same claims were printed in an oft-quoted (in this context, too-oft-quoted) academic paper.[25] During the COVID-19 pandemic, this association has been repeated so often that it seems self-evident.

CUI BONO, CUI MALO

Journalists have their own reasons for mentioning Mary. Medical researchers, in turn, might throw in her name as a historical seasoning to a paper, as a preemptive step against the unavoidable request from "Reviewer2" ("Mention Mary!"), or to suggest that there is epidemiological evidence, going back 110 years, that some people—or, people under certain circumstances—can become especially dangerous and efficient disseminators of pathogenic agents. Public health officials might also believe that reference to a well-known story could help convey better the idea that ignoring the instructions of medical authorities might lead to disastrous consequences.

Educating the public on the need to follow medical instructions, especially during an epidemic, is in itself a noble cause. Uncritically invoking Mary's name for that purpose, however, is probably counterproductive. For what Mary's story truly brings to the surface is a long legacy of stigmatizing people by signaling them out as health dangers. Invoking Mary means shifting the focus, the responsibility, and perhaps also the blame from the level of the state or municipality to that of the (unruly) individuals, or to the classes of people to which they belong. In this latter sense, too, the figure of Typhoid Mary sets a very bad example for how public health causes should be advanced by medical professionals.

In other words, the greatest problem with associating Mary with the concept of super-spreader is not that it is anachronistic (projecting contemporary concepts and concerns into the past), nor that airborne viruses and gastrointestinal bacteria are different types of pathogens, nor even that various mistakes creeped into the description of Mary's epidemiological harm. The problem with this association is that references to Mary as a super-spreader are inadvertently bidirectional. They do not only imply that Mary was a super-spreader but also that those who are found today to have been "super-spreaders" are "Typhoid Marys"—human manifestations of disease, immanent dangers to society, and at least partially responsible, because of their negligent hygienic behavior or ignorance, for the infections that they cause. During the COVID-19 pandemic, public discussion on "super-spreaders" was all-too-often accompanied by racial and religious antagonism, gendered stereotypes, and hate speech directed at certain groups—political opponents, minorities, foreigners, or lower classes. Doctors would do well to excise discriminatory overtones from professional discourse. Unless their explicit intention is to critically unpack Mary's story, it might be a good time to finally lay her to rest. AJPH

CORRESPONDENCE

Correspondence should be sent to Amir Teicher, Department of History, Faculty of Humanities, Tel Aviv University, Tel Aviv 6997801, Israel (e-mail: teichera@tauex.tau.ac.il). Reprints can be ordered at https://ajph.org by clicking the "Reprints" link.

PUBLICATION INFORMATION

Full Citation: Teicher A. Typhoid Mary was not a super-spreader (and super-spreaders are not "Typhoid Marys"). *Am J Public Health*. 2023;113(12): 1249–1253.

Acceptance Date: August 27, 2023.

DOI: https://doi.org/10.2105/AJPH.2023.307434

ACKNOWLEDGMENTS

The Tel Aviv University Center for Combatting Pandemics, the Alexander von Humboldt Stiftung, the Institute for the History of Medicine at Giessen University, and the Max Planck Institute for the History of Science provided financial and institutional support for this research.

I thank Basmat Kislev for her assistance and Sarah Mandel for her proofreading.

CONFLICTS OF INTEREST

No conflicts of interest are declared.

REFERENCES

1. Leavitt JW. *Typhoid Mary: Captive to the Public's Health*. Boston, MA: Beacon Press; 1997.
2. Ogan ML. Immunization in a typhoid outbreak in the Sloane Hospital for Women. *N Y State J Med*. 1915;101:610–612.
3. Sawyer WA. The efficacy of various anti-typhoid vaccines. *J Am Med Assoc*. 1915;LXV(17):1413–1418. https://doi.org/10.1001/jama.1915.02580170001001
4. Mystery of the poison guest at wealthy Mrs. Case's party. *The San Francisco Examiner*. August 29, 1920: 68.
5. Death at the wedding feast. *The San Francisco Examiner*. June 28, 1931: 83.
6. Sultan L, Nyka W, Mills C, O'Grady F, Riley RL, Wells W. Tuberculosis disseminators: a study of the variability of aerial infectivity of tuberculous patients. *Am Rev Respir Dis*. 1960;82(3):358–369. https://doi.org/10.1164/arrd.1960.82.3.358
7. Schulman JL, Kilbourne ED. Experimental transmission of influenza virus infection in mice: II. Some factors affecting the incidence of transmitted infection. *J Exp Med*. 1963;118(2):267–275. https://doi.org/10.1084/jem.118.2.267
8. Gerone PJ, Couch RB, Keefer GV, Douglas RG, Derrenbacher EB, Knight V. Assessment of experimental and natural viral aerosols. *Bacteriol Rev*. 1966;30(3):576–588. https://doi.org/10.1128/br.30.3.576-588.1966
9. Fox JP, Kilbourne ED. Epidemiology of influenza: summary of influenza workshop IV. *J Infect Dis*. 1973;128(3):361–386. https://doi.org/10.1093/infdis/128.3.361
10. Osborn SH, Beckler EA. Once a typhoid carrier, always a typhoid carrier. *J Infect Dis*. 1920;27(2):145–150. https://doi.org/10.1093/infdis/27.2.145
11. Chapin CV. *The Sources and Modes of Infection*. New York, NY: John Wiley & Sons; 1916.
12. Wald P. *Contagious: Cultures, Carriers, and the Outbreak Narrative*. Durham, NC: Duke University Press; 2008.
13. Soper GA. Typhoid Mary. *TSG*. 1919;45(1):1–15.

14. Treadway WL. The laboratory in relation to the control of communicable diseases. *Ir J Med Sci.* 1927;2(12):721–725. https://doi.org/10.1007/BF02960693
15. Rosenau MJ. *Preventive Medicine and Hygiene.* New York, NY: D. Appleton; 1921.
16. Jones GW. The scourge of typhoid. *Am Hist Illus.* 1967;1:22–28.
17. Stafford J. Psittacosis Polly—more menacing than Typhoid Mary. *Asbury Park Sunday Press.* February 12, 1939: 11.
18. Talley R. 'Memphis' 25 'Typhoid Marys' walk streets laden with billions of germs. *The Commercial Appeal Memphis.* January 25, 1948: 39.
19. State battles 'Typhoid Marys,' carriers of citrus killing virus. *The Sacramento Bee.* June 3, 1963: 17.
20. Winter R. Psychotic Typhoid Mary's help spread mental disease. *The Amarillo Globe-Times.* December 9, 1965: 28.
21. Anderson RM, May RM. Population Biology of Infectious Diseases: Report of the Dahlem Workshop on Population Biology of Infectious Disease Agents, Berlin, 1982, March 14–19. Berlin, Germany: Springer; 1982.
22. May RM. The impact, transmission, and evolution of infectious diseases. *Nature.* 1982;297(5867):539–540. https://doi.org/10.1038/297539a0
23. Khamsi R. Could sneeze meters combat pandemics? *Nature.* November 16, 2005. https://doi.org/10.1038/news051114-7
24. Hudson PJ, Perkins SE, Cattadori IM. The emergence of wildlife disease and the application of ecology. In: Ostfeld RS, Keesing F, Eviner VT, eds. *Infectious Disease Ecology: Effects of Ecosystems on Disease and of Disease on Ecosystems.* Princeton, NJ: Princeton University Press; 2008: 347–367.
25. Marineli F, Tsoucalas G, Karamanou M, Androutsos G. Mary Mallon (1869–1938) and the history of typhoid fever. *Ann Gastroenterol.* 2013;26(2):132–134.

A Medicaid-Funded Statewide Diabetes Quality Improvement Collaborative: Ohio 2020–2022

Shari D. Bolen, MD, MPH, Joshua J. Joseph, MD, MPH, Kathleen M. Dungan, MD, MPH, Elizabeth A. Beverly, PhD, Adam T. Perzynski, PhD, Douglas Einstadter, MD, MPH, Jordan Fiegl, MS, Thomas E. Love, PhD, Douglas Spence, PhD, Katherine Jenkins, MPH, Allison Lorenz, MPA, Shah Jalal Uddin, MS, MA, Kelly McCutcheon Adams, MSW, LICSW, Michael W. Konstan, MD, and Mary S. Applegate, MD, on behalf of the Diabetes Quality Improvement Collaborative

We used a collective impact model to form a statewide diabetes quality improvement collaborative to improve diabetes outcomes and advance diabetes health equity. Between 2020 and 2022, in collaboration with the Ohio Department of Medicaid, Medicaid Managed Care Plans, and Ohio's seven medical schools, we recruited 20 primary care practices across the state. The percentage of patients with hemoglobin A1c greater than 9% improved from 25% to 20% over two years. Applying our model more broadly could accelerate improvement in diabetes outcomes. (*Am J Public Health*. 2023;113(12): 1254–1257. https://doi.org/10.2105/AJPH.2023.307410)

AJPH December 2023, Vol 113, No. 12

To improve hemoglobin A1c (A1c) levels and reduce the rate of complications and costs for Medicaid enrollees with diabetes,[1] the Ohio Department of Medicaid partnered with the Ohio Colleges of Medicine Government Resource Center, Medicaid Managed Care Plans (MCPs), and the seven Ohio medical schools to develop a statewide diabetes collaborative focused on improving diabetes outcomes and advancing diabetes health equity.

INTERVENTION AND IMPLEMENTATION

Partners participated in a planning year using the collective impact model as a mechanism for shared power to address complex challenges.[2] The collective impact model[2] has five key elements:

1. a common agenda (i.e., shared vision, mission and project aims),
2. shared measurement (i.e., electronic health record [EHR] data queries),
3. mutually reinforcing activities (i.e., intervention and implementation strategies),
4. continuous communication (i.e., routine steering committee meetings every two weeks), and
5. backbone support (i.e., organizational structure and roles for all partners).

During this year, we also developed a key driver diagram and toolkit to reflect the theory for improvement and guide the quality improvement (QI) activities.[3]

Partners recruited 20 primary care practices across 11 health systems to participate in the QI project. All participating practices served a high volume of Medicaid patients, and health systems were given $25 000 in stipends to submit EHR data. The overall aim of the QI project was to decrease the percentage of adults with diabetes with A1c greater than 9% from 25% to 21% overall. To supplement the QI activities, the Ohio Department of Medicaid requested that the six MCPs align their QI projects with the activities of the QI practices to catalyze improvements in outcomes over time. In response to barriers to diabetes care voiced by providers and patients, Medicaid payers added coverage for Diabetes Self-Management Education and Support, three payers removed prior authorization requirements for continuous glucose monitors, and all payers aligned quantity limits on diabetes supplies and piloted home A1c testing. These MCP interventions enhanced equity to Medicaid enrollees by making it easier to obtain and afford diabetes supplies and resources, especially during the COVID-19 pandemic.

Implementation strategies included audit and feedback, peer-to-peer learning, QI coaching, and subject matter expert consultation. After the planning year, a half-day virtual kick off was held with the participating primary care practices, Medicaid MCPs, and other partners. This was followed by monthly QI coaching calls with each of the practices and monthly one-hour webinars or "action period calls" with the practices and MCPs to share aggregate practice-level data, discuss evidence-based best practices, and promote peer-to-peer learning. In addition, there were two virtual learning sessions held to increase peer-to-peer learning. Lastly, we held monthly one-hour collaborative calls with the MCPs and a subset of clinical practices and partners to enhance their collaborative planning.

Practices submitted EHR data every two weeks to the Ohio Colleges of Medicine Government Resource Center, which developed an online dashboard for practices to monitor progress when conducting continuous QI. Key interventions tested by the practices included (1) A1c testing for those with no test within the last 12 months, (2) timely follow-up in team-based care—defined as follow-up scheduled virtually or in person with a primary care provider or team member (e.g., a clinical pharmacist, dietitian, or diabetes educator) at least every 30 days until the glucose level was at goal, (3) outreach to re-engage patients with A1c greater than 9% and no upcoming appointment, and (4) social drivers of health interventions (e.g., community health worker engagement, referrals to resources for healthy food, mobile vans, or virtual care).

PLACE, TIME, AND PERSONS

The QI project started in June 2020, with the previous 12 months considered the preintervention period (June 1, 2019, to May 31, 2020). Hence, year 1 of the QI project extended from June 1, 2020, through April 2021, and year 2 extended from May 1, 2021, to June 30, 2022. We included a total of 35 151 patients with type 2 diabetes. We included patients with type 2 diabetes identified from the EHR using *International Classification of Diseases, Ninth Revision, Clinical Modification* (Hyattsville, MD: National Center for Health Statistics; 1980) codes 250.0–250.9, 357.2, 362.0, and 366.41 and *International Classification of Diseases, 10th Revision* (Geneva, Switzerland: World Health Organization; 1992) codes E10.0–E14.9. The mean age of patients with diabetes was 56.7 (SD = 14.7) years, 52.8% were female, 48.4% had hypertension, and 25% had baseline A1c greater than 9%. Self-reported race/ethnicity was 47.0% White, 38.9% non-Hispanic Black, 7.4% Hispanic, and 6.7% other, and the primary insurance type was 39.6% Medicare, 27.4% Medicaid, 31.1% commercial, and 1.9% uninsured or self-pay.

PURPOSE

Our primary aim was to align primary care practices and MCPs to improve diabetes health outcomes, with a specific initial focus on improving A1c levels.

EVALUATION AND ADVERSE EFFECTS

We evaluated the QI project impact using the following aggregated measures: (1) A1c tested in the last 12 months for all patients with diabetes, (2) follow-up visit scheduled virtually or in person if A1c was greater than 9%, and (3) most recent A1c greater than 9% (primary outcome). We measured outcomes longitudinally using repeated cross-sections of EHR data and presented results as statistical process control charts with upper and lower confidence limits. We placed a shift in the mean when eight consecutive points were above the upper confidence limit on the control chart, and this corresponded to a new intervention implemented at the practices according to the methodologies set forth in *The Health Care Data Guide*.[4] We used three times the standard deviation as the confidence limits.

We did not have a balancing measure to determine adverse effects because all other EHR measures had some relation to diabetes care, although these measures like depression screening improved or stayed the same indicating no clear adverse effect (data not shown).

Figure 1 demonstrates that adults with diabetes and A1c greater than 9% seen at the primary care practices improved from 25% at baseline to 20% by the end of the intervention. A1c levels worsened initially during the COVID-19 pandemic, returned to baseline, and then improved beyond baseline as the practices were able to implement protocols to improve glycemic control in the context of COVID-19. Figures A and B (available as supplements to the online version of this article at https://ajph.org) demonstrate the process improvements in A1c testing and scheduled follow-up in team-based care. We were unable to measure processes related to social drivers of health interventions and MCP interventions because of the challenges in capturing these data.

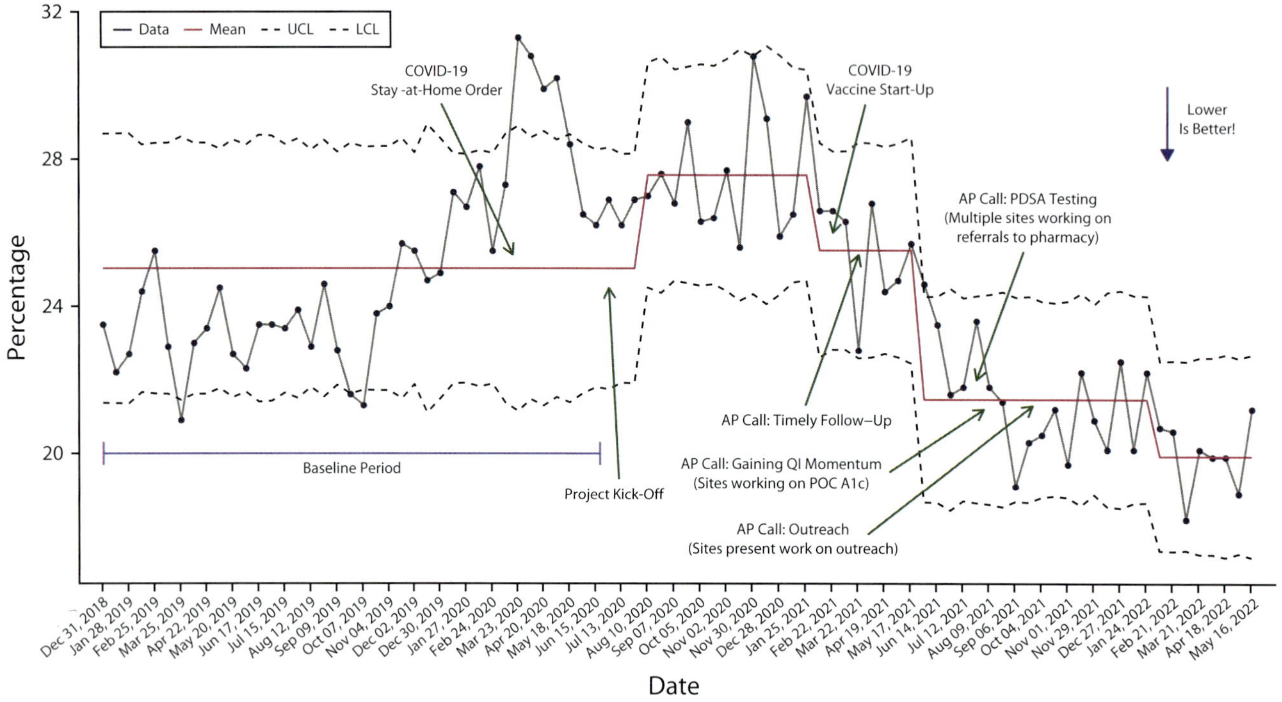

FIGURE 1— Percentage of Adults With Diabetes Whose Most Recent Hemoglobin A1c Was Greater Than 9% for All Sites Combined by Month: Ohio, 2020–2022

Note. AP = action period call or webinar; LCL = lower confidence limit; PDSA = plan, do, study, act; POC A1c = point of care A1c testing; QI = quality improvement; UCL = upper confidence limit. Monthly sample size: median = 1730; minimum = 1099; maximum = 2361.

SUSTAINABILITY

As a mechanism for sustaining gains and for larger spread across Medicaid enrollees, the Ohio Department of Medicaid is currently funding regional QI hubs at each of the seven medical schools and encouraging recruitment of 10 to 25 practices initially in each region, with an eventual goal of reaching at least 50% of Medicaid enrollees in each of the seven regions. Data on whether practices were able to maintain gains were not captured and were outside the scope of this project. However, similar implementation strategies within the context of a regional QI collaborative led to sustained improvements in blood pressure control for more than two years.[5,6]

PUBLIC HEALTH SIGNIFICANCE

At a time of great chaos within health care associated with worsening of chronic conditions because of COVID-19,[7] we succeeded in establishing a statewide diabetes QI collaborative to improve A1c control in patients with diabetes at primary care practices with a high volume of Medicaid enrollees throughout Ohio. Using evidence-based data-driven interventions tailored to the practice and patient is essential for successful large-scale QI efforts in primary care. While many QI efforts for diabetes have been successful, there are no statewide models for diabetes improvement. A statewide model avoids policy barriers that may exist across states for payers and health care systems and has the potential for larger benefit than regional approaches within a state. This model for statewide health improvement for populations with a high volume of Medicaid enrollees could be expanded within a state by using medical schools or other trusted clinical and QI organizations. AJPH

ABOUT THE AUTHORS

Shari D. Bolen is with the Department of Medicine, The MetroHealth Medical Center and Case Western Reserve University, Cleveland, OH. Joshua J. Joseph is with the Department of Internal Medicine, The Ohio State University Wexner Medical Center, Columbus. Kathleen M. Dungan is with the Department of Medicine, The Ohio State University Wexner Medical Center, Columbus. Elizabeth A. Beverly is with the Department of Primary Care at The Diabetes Institute, Ohio University, Athens. Adam T. Perzynski is with the Department of Medicine and Department of Sociology, The MetroHealth Medical Center and Case Western Reserve

University. Douglas Einstadter and Jordan Fiegl are with the Department of Medicine, The MetroHealth Medical Center and Case Western Reserve University. Thomas E. Love is with the Department of Medicine and Population and Quantitative Health Sciences, The MetroHealth Medical Center and Case Western Reserve University. Douglas Spence, Katherine Jenkins, Allison Lorenz, and Shah Jalal Uddin are with The Ohio State Government Resource Center, Columbus. Kelly McCutcheon Adams is with the Institute for Healthcare Improvement, Boston, MA. Michael W. Konstan is with the Department of Pediatrics, Case Western Reserve University. Mary S. Applegate is with the Ohio Department of Medicaid, Columbus.

CORRESPONDENCE

Correspondence should be sent to Shari D. Bolen, MD, MPH, 2500 MetroHealth Drive, Rammelkamp Building, R220A, Cleveland, OH 44109 (e-mail: sbolen@metrohealth.org). Reprints can be ordered at https://ajph.org by clicking the "Reprints" link.

PUBLICATION INFORMATION

Full Citation: Bolen SD, Joseph JJ, Dungan KM, et al. A Medicaid-funded statewide diabetes quality improvement collaborative: Ohio 2020–2022. *Am J Public Health*. 2023;113(12):1254–1257.

Acceptance Date: August 1, 2023.

DOI: https://doi.org/10.2105/AJPH.2023.307410

CONTRIBUTORS

S. D. Bolen and J. J. Joseph were involved in project design, implementation, data analysis and interpretation, and writing and revising the article. K. M. Dungan, E. A. Beverly, A. T. Perzynski, K. Jenkins, A. Lorenz, K. M. Adams, and M. S. Applegate were involved in project design, implementation, data analysis interpretation, and critically revising the article. D. Einstadter was involved in project design; implementation; data extraction, analysis, and interpretation; and critically revising the article. J. Fiegl was involved in data analysis and interpretation, and in writing and critically revising the article. T. E. Love was involved in project design, data analysis and interpretation, and critically revising the article. D. Spence and S. J. Uddin were involved in data extraction, analysis, and interpretation, and in critically revising the article. M. W. Konstan was involved in project design, data analysis interpretation, and critically revising the article.

ACKNOWLEDGMENTS

Funding for the Diabetes Quality Improvement (QI) project was provided by the Ohio Department of Medicaid's Medicaid Technical Assistance and Policy Program.

We have previously presented aspects of this project at the National Society of General Internal Medicine Conference 2022 and Academy Health's Annual Research Meeting 2023.

The authors gratefully acknowledge the administrative support of the Ohio Colleges of Medicine Government Resources Center and partnership of the Ohio Department of Medicaid, Ohio Medicaid Managed Care Plans, Ohio medical schools, QI consultants, and primary care clinics throughout Ohio.

Note. The authors are solely responsible for this article's contents, findings, and conclusions, which do not represent the views of the state of Ohio, Ohio Department of Medicaid (ODM), or any federal programs. Readers should not interpret any statement in this report as an official position of ODM or of Health and Human Services.

CONFLICTS OF INTEREST

K. M. Dungan discloses research support from Sanofi, Viacyte, Abbott, and Dexcom; consulting with Eli Lilly and Dexcom; and honoraria from UptoDate, Elsevier, Med Learning Group, Medscape, and Cardiometabolic Health Congress.

HUMAN PARTICIPANT PROTECTION

While the Diabetes QI Project was deemed not human participant research, we did have an institutional review board (IRB) and data use agreement to evaluate the retrospective electronic health record data from the project at Case Western Reserve University under IRB STUDY20191098.

REFERENCES

1. Centers for Medicare and Medicaid Services. Comprehensive diabetes care: hemoglobin A1c (HbA1c) poor control (>9.0%): ages 18 to 75. Available at: https://www.medicaid.gov/state-overviews/scorecard/comprehensive-diabetes-care/index.html. Accessed February 25, 2023.
2. Kania J, Kramer M. Collective impact. *Stanf Soc Innov Rev.* 2011;9(1) 36–41. https://doi.org/10.48558/5900-KN19
3. Bolen SD, Beverly EA, Khoury S, et al. Forming Cardi-OH: a statewide collaborative to improve cardiovascular health in Ohio. *Cureus.* 2022;14(8):e28381. https://doi.org/10.7759/cureus.28381
4. Provost L, Murray S. *The Health Care Data Guide: Learning From Data for Improvement.* Hoboken, NJ: John Wiley & Sons; 2011.
5. Pfoh ER, Martinez K, Vakharia N, Rothberg M. Impact of a system-wide quality improvement initiative on blood pressure control: a cohort analysis. *BMJ Qual Saf.* 2020;29(3):225–231. https://doi.org/10.1136/bmjqs-2018-009032
6. Bolen SD, Love TE, Einstadter D, et al. Improving regional blood pressure control: a positive deviance tiered intensity approach. *J Gen Intern Med.* 2021;36(6):1591–1597. https://doi.org/10.1007/s11606-020-06480-z
7. Nielsen VM, Song G, Ojamaa LS, Blodgett RP, Rocchio CM, Pennock JN. The COVID-19 pandemic and access to selected ambulatory care services among populations with severely uncontrolled diabetes and hypertension in Massachusetts. *Public Health Rep.* 2022;137(2):344–351. https://doi.org/10.1177/00333549211065515

Countering Mpox Vaccination Disparities in Los Angeles County, California, May–December 2022

Auguste Brihn, DVM, MPH, Nava Yeganeh, MD, MPH, Sonali Kulkarni, MD, MPH, Olivia Moir, MSc, Saloniki Madrid, MA, Mario Perez, MPH, Rita Singhal, MD, MPH, and Andrea A. Kim, PhD, MPH

Providing equitable access to vaccines for individuals at risk for mpox was critical for containing the 2022 mpox outbreak in Los Angeles County, California. Eligible non-Hispanic Black/African American and Latinx individuals had lower vaccine uptake than did non-Hispanic White individuals, despite having higher mpox case rates. Strategies to address disparities in vaccine uptake included using familiar messaging technology to reach individuals at risk for mpox, using partnerships with community-based organizations to raise mpox awareness, and bringing vaccines to locations convenient to at-risk individuals to improve access. (*Am J Public Health*. 2023;113(12):1258–1262. https://doi.org/10.2105/AJPH.2023.307409)

AJPH December 2023, Vol 113, No. 12

On May 19, 2022, the first case of mpox was identified in Los Angeles County (LAC), California.[1] In response to the outbreak, the LAC Department of Public Health (LACDPH) implemented a phased strategy to manage the limited vaccine supply made available through the Federal Strategic National Stockpile for persons at risk for mpox.[2] The combination of low supply and high demand for vaccines revealed inequities in vaccine access and uptake, with lower vaccine rates among Latinx and non-Hispanic Black/African American individuals despite having higher mpox case rates than did non-Hispanic White individuals.

INTERVENTION AND IMPLEMENTATION

To address these disparities, we implemented interventions that were guided by lessons learned from the COVID-19 vaccine response in Los Angeles County. These interventions included (1) increasing access for individuals with recent sexually transmitted infections through text-messaging campaigns (per Title 17, California Code of Regulations, section 2500(b), syphilis and gonorrhea are reportable to LACDPH); (2) establishing vaccine partnerships with a geographically dispersed network of community providers (i.e., HIV Pre-Exposure Prophylaxis Centers of Excellence and Ryan White Program–supported HIV specialty federally qualified health clinics, hospitals, LACDPH public vaccination sites, and pharmacies); (3) bringing vaccines to convenient locations, including pop-up clinics at community events for non-Hispanic Black/African American men who have sex with men (MSM), Latinx MSM, and the transgender community; Pride events celebrating Lesbian, Gay, Bisexual, Transgender, Queer or Questioning, Asexual, Intersex, and Others (LGBTQAI+) culture and rights; MSM nightclubs; and commercial sex venues; and (4) communicating with providers through weekly office hours and recurring situational update meetings with Latinx MSM, non-Hispanic Black/African American MSM, and transgender community stakeholders (i.e., activists, clinical staff, community-based organizations, and academic partners). These meetings included a discussion of strategies to address vaccine confidence in these communities.[3]

PLACE, TIME, AND PERSONS

LAC has a population of nearly 10 million residents,[4] spans more than 4000 square miles, and is marked by diversity in race/ethnicity, language, culture, and socioeconomic status, making widespread and equitable access to vaccines challenging.

At the outbreak onset, an estimated 120 000 residents were at risk for mpox. We defined the population at risk as persons at increased risk for mpox exposure and recommended to receive the vaccine. We applied a standardized Centers for Disease Control and Prevention formula to estimate the size of the at-risk population.[5] This included the number of MSM living with diagnosed HIV and the estimated number of MSM eligible for HIV preexposure prophylaxis. We increased the sum of these by 25% to account for additional vaccine-eligible people not captured in these two groups. We estimated vaccine coverage by dividing the number of people vaccinated with one dose and two doses by the estimated size of the at-risk population. Despite the large number of residents who could benefit from vaccination, LAC's strategy required phased expansion of vaccine eligibility to balance limited supply and reach the highest risk groups (Table A, available as a supplement to the online version of this article at http://www.ajph.org). Initially, vaccines were prioritized for persons confirmed to have either a high- or intermediate-risk contact to an mpox case. Vaccine eligibility expanded as more vaccines became available through phases 1 through 4 of the National Monkeypox Vaccine Strategy.

Phase 1 supply enabled vaccines to be offered to persons confirmed to have attended large social events also attended by persons with confirmed infection; however, this supply could only potentially reach an estimated 5% of the at-risk population. Phases 2 and 3 vaccines allowed greater coverage of at-risk individuals by expanding access to persons who self-attested to being gay, bisexual, or other MSM or transgender persons and had (1) rectal gonorrhea or early syphilis in the past three months, (2) multiple or anonymous sex partners in the past 14 days, or (3) skin-to-skin contact at a large venue or event in the past 14 days. Phase 4 vaccination provided sufficient supply to widen vaccine eligibility to any man or transgender person who had sex with men or transgender persons, persons of any gender or sexual orientation who engaged in commercial or transactional sex, persons living with HIV, sexual partners of people listed, and any person who anticipated being in any of the groups listed. By December 22, 2022, we removed all eligibility requirements, and the vaccine became available to anyone requesting it.

PURPOSE

As phase 1 launched, LACDPH partnered with HIV Pre-Exposure Prophylaxis Centers of Excellence and Ryan White Program–supported HIV specialty clinics to offer vaccines to patients who met phase 1 eligibility criteria. Beginning July 17, 2022, LACDPH supplemented these efforts by offering vaccines at LACDPH-operated mass vaccination sites (Figure A, available as a supplement to the online version of this article at http://www.ajph.org). However, accessing vaccines at these larger public sites required access to high-speed Internet to preregister for vaccine, a cellphone that received texts to confirm vaccine availability, and transportation to vaccination sites, which favored individuals living with more resources. By the end of July 2022, disparities in vaccination uptake began to emerge. Although 40% of mpox cases were among Latinx individuals, only 31% of doses were administered to Latinx individuals. Similarly, non-Hispanic Black/African American individuals represented 11% of cases but only received 8% of doses. By contrast, 46% of vaccines were administered to non-Hispanic White individuals, although they only comprised 29% of cases. These disparities in vaccine uptake challenged LACDPH to identify barriers faced by Latinx and non-Hispanic Black/African American MSM and improve vaccination opportunities for these groups.

EVALUATION AND ADVERSE EFFECTS

By December 2022, LAC providers administered 116 629 doses of vaccine, covering an estimated 60% of the at-risk population with partial vaccination (one dose) and 35% with full vaccination (two doses). With the arrival of more vaccines in phase 2, eligibility was updated to enable more people to be vaccinated. Simultaneously, provider vaccine capacity at "fixed sites" (e.g., clinic and pharmacy locations) and mobile vaccine pop-up clinics in the community expanded. In phase 2, LACDPH implemented an online vaccine registration portal allowing individuals to sign up for vaccines starting on July 20, 2022. Immediately following these activities, we observed a sevenfold increase in vaccines administered from the week of July 11 to July 25 (Figure A), including a ninefold increase among Latinx residents and a sevenfold increase among non-Hispanic Black/African American individuals.

Despite improved vaccine access, we observed disparities in vaccination rates among non-Hispanic Black/African American and Latinx individuals, prompting rapid interventions to be designed for these groups. Starting in September 2022, LACDPH implemented a series of targeted pop-up vaccine clinics and promotional events in partnership with community organizations that serve Latinx and non-Hispanic Black/African American at-risk individuals. By year-end 2022, 40% of newly vaccinated persons each week were Latinx and 12% were non-Hispanic Black/African American (Figure 1).

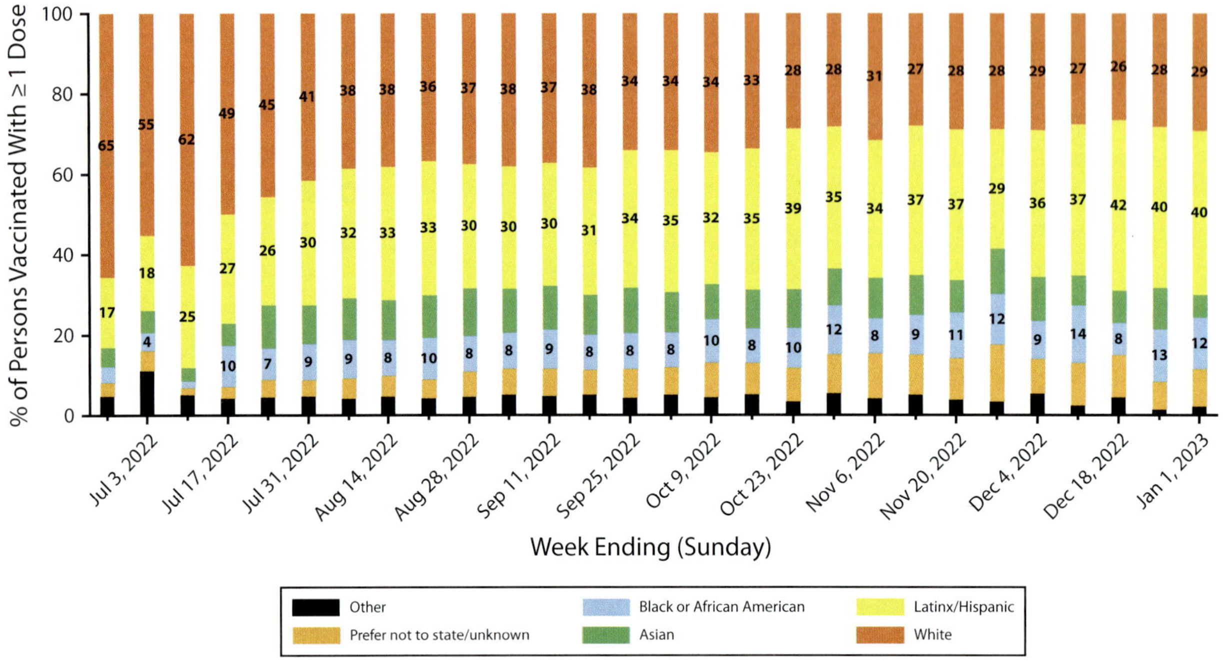

FIGURE 1— Racial/Ethnic Distribution Among Persons Who Received a First Dose of JYNNEOS Vaccine by Week: Los Angeles County, California, July–December 2022

Note. JYNNEOS is the brand name used in the United States for Bavarian Nordic's (Hellerup, Denmark) MVA-BN (modified vaccinia Ankara–Bavarian Nordic) vaccine.

TABLE 1— Weekly Distribution of Race/Ethnicity Among Persons Receiving One or More Doses of JYNNEOS by First-Dose Provider: Los Angeles County, California, May–December 2022

	First-Dose Vaccine Provider Type					
Race/ Ethnicity	**Public Health,[a] No. (%)**	**Mobile Vaccine Team/ Pharmacy,[b] No. (%)**	**Community Clinic,[c] No. (%)**	**Health System,[d] No. (%)**	**Unknown, No. (%)**	**Total, No. (%)**
Latinx	10 091 (29.7)	3 448 (25.5)	7 331 (36.9)	1 860 (40.6)	18 (36.0)	22 730 (31.6)
Asian	3 932 (11.6)	1 437 (10.6)	1 638 (8.3)	414 (9.0)	≤5 (. . .)	7 421 (10.3)
Non-Hispanic Black/African American	2 844 (8.4)	932 (6.9)	2 261 (11.4)	576 (12.6)	≤5 (. . .)	6 613 (9.2)
Non-Hispanic White	13 828 (40.7)	5 998 (44.4)	6 725 (33.9)	1 319 (28.8)	19 (38.0)	27 870 (38.7)
Other[e]	1 617 (4.8)	617 (4.6)	818 (4.1)	228 (5.0)	≤5 (. . .)	3 280 (4.6)
Unknown	1 705 (5.0)	1 077 (8.0)	1 080 (5.4)	186 (4.1)	≤5 (. . .)	4 048 (5.6)
Total	34 017 (100.0)	13 509 (100.0)	19 853 (100.0)	4 583 (100.0)	50 (100.0)	71 962 (100.0)

Note. LAC = Los Angeles County. Sample size was n = 71 962. JYNNEOS is the brand name used in the United States for Bavarian Nordic's (Hellerup, Denmark) MVA-BN (modified vaccinia Ankara–Bavarian Nordic) vaccine. Percentages may not add to 100% because of rounding.

[a]Vaccines administered at the Department of Public Health points of distribution or mass vaccinations sites.
[b]Department of Public Health mobile vaccine teams or providers contracted by mobile vaccine teams. Pharmacies were included in this category because they administered most of their doses at pop-up clinics and were funded by LAC Department of Public Health as mobile vaccine teams.
[c]Any non-LAC Department of Public Health clinic providing public mpox vaccinations, including community providers.
[d]Group health care organizations and hospital systems in LAC.
[e]Other race includes American Indian/Alaska Native, Native Hawaiian/other Pacific Islander, multiracial, and persons reporting other race. Unknown race includes persons who reported they preferred not to state their race/ethnicity and other persons with unknown race/ethnicity.

Importantly, HIV and sexually transmitted infection community clinics that offered mpox vaccines demonstrated that they could reach higher percentages of Latinx and non-Hispanic Black/African American at-risk individuals than could other vaccine providers (Table 1), most likely because they were trusted entities in the LGBTQIA+ community.

SUSTAINABILITY

At the outbreak's onset, LACDPH recruited providers at trusted community locations to administer vaccines. Using lessons learned from the local COVID-19 vaccine response, these provider efforts were supplemented with mass public vaccination sites to meet the large community demand. The longstanding relationships between LACDPH and LGBTQIA+ community partners helped to rapidly establish a robust vaccine provider network that was accessible to persons who would benefit most from vaccination. In addition, engagement of community leaders and providers through regular stakeholder briefings provided a space to exchange information on outbreak trends, transmission risk, and vaccine updates as the outbreak evolved. Prompt access to information helped address common misconceptions and concerns about vaccination. It also allowed familiar and entrusted community partners to message mpox vaccine information to help reduce stigma and misinformation. Maintaining these community-driven partnerships across LAC was needed for LACDPH to respond effectively to the mpox outbreak and is a sustainable and equitable model for responding to future vaccine preventable disease outbreaks in highly affected groups.

PUBLIC HEALTH SIGNIFICANCE

Ensuring that all individuals have access to vaccines is a priority for preventing a resurgence of mpox. Strategic engagement with a diverse range of community providers, agile vaccine clinic models, and familiar information technology tools are needed to reach the right populations and address disparities in vaccine access. A strong public health partnership with public and private health care providers should be maintained to ensure a rapid, accessible, and equitable response to public health emergencies. AJPH

ABOUT THE AUTHORS

Auguste Brihn, Nava Yeganeh, Olivia Moir, Saloniki Madrid, Rita Singhal, and Andrea A. Kim are with the Vaccine Preventable Disease Control Program, Los Angeles County Department of Public Health, Los Angeles, CA. Sonali Kulkarni and Mario Perez are with the Division of HIV and STD Programs, Los Angeles County Department of Public Health.

CORRESPONDENCE

Correspondence should be sent to Nava Yeganeh, MD, MPH, 3530 Wilshire Blvd #700, Los Angeles, CA 90010 (e-mail: nyeganeh@ph.lacounty.gov). Reprints can be ordered at http://www.ajph.org by clicking the "Reprints" link.

PUBLICATION INFORMATION

Full Citation: Brihn A, Yeganeh N, Kulkarni S, et al. Countering mpox vaccination disparities in Los Angeles County, California, May–December 2022. *Am J Public Health*. 2023;113(12):1258–1262.

Acceptance Date: August 1, 2023.

DOI: https://doi.org/10.2105/AJPH.2023.307409

CONTRIBUTORS

A. Brihn, N. Yeganeh, O. Moir, and A. A. Kim conceptualized and visualized the article and wrote the first draft. N. Yeganeh, S. Kulkarni, M. Perez, R. Singhal, and A. A. Kim conceptualized the public health intervention. O. Moir provided data analysis and visualization. All authors contributed to data validation, edited the article, and wrote the final draft.

ACKNOWLEDGMENTS

This article and the authors' work were supported by the Centers for Disease Control and Prevention (CDC) of the US Department of Health and Human Services (HHS) as part of a financial assistance award totaling $65,864,224.00 with 100% funded by the CDC.

The Los Angeles County Department of Public Health Mpox Vaccine Operations Team aided in this work: Dee Ann Bagwell, Sharon Balter, Melanie Barr, Sandra Buenrrostro, Wendi Cate, Alex Choo, Adriana Diaz, Christine Erinakis, Laurel Fowler, Natalie Frey, Daniel Hancz, Laurie Hensley-Wojcieszyn, Courtney Jones, Jee Kim, Jennifer Lee, Aizita Magana, Cristin Mondy, Maria Mongiardo, Kim Moore, Leo Moore, Gema Morales-Meyer, Janina Morrison, Emy Murakami, Amanda Nguyen, Sandra Perez, Annie Pham, Devon Rax, Shelby Redman, Tiffany Romo, Carissa Sepulveda, Erick Serrano, Naman Shah, Aseniq Shahid-Williams, Michelle Shishkin, Lucy Stillman, Matthew Tecle, Dawn Terashita, Lello Tesema, Jasmine Ting, Dulmini Wilson, Jessica Woodard, Marc Yang, and Sherry Yin. Additional data support was provided by James Beekley, Max Camacho, Elmer Carmagopena, Kenneth Chapin, Jonathan Chang, Nicholas Crouch, Phoebe Danza, Christine Erinakis, Rebecca Fisher, Natalie Frey, Megan Halbrook, Bianca Katnik, Marena Lin, Maria Mongiardo, Syeda Naqvi, Erin Nguyen, Kathleen Poortinga, Benjamin Scott, Charles Strauber, and Thanga Gabby Darshana Suthakar. We would also like to thank all the mpox vaccine providers throughout Los Angeles County: 986 Pharmacy, Access to Prevention and Advocacy Intervention, AIDS Healthcare Foundation, All Inclusive Community Health Center, Alondra Pharmacy, Altamed Medical Group, Arleta Urgent Care, APLA Health and Wellness, ASPIRE RX, Inc., Cal Poly Pomona, Ambulnz Health, LLC, Bartz-Altadonna Community Health Center, Bienestar Human Services, Capital Drugs, Aviva Pharmacy, California State University Long Beach Student Health, Central Neighborhood Health Foundation, City of Long Beach Department of Health and Human Services, City of Pasadena Public Health Department, Clinica Familiar San Lucas, CHAP Med, Children's Hospital Los Angeles, Clinica Monsenor Oscar A Romero, Correctional Health Services, Cosmed Pharmacy, East Valley Community Health Center, DeNovo Health Care, Dripology, El Monte Pharmacy, El Proyecto Del Barrio, Elements Pharmacy, Fatima Medical Clinic, Fulgent Genetics, Garfield Health Center, El Camino College Student Health Services, Family Health Care Resources, Infectious Disease Specialists of Long Beach, JWCH Institute, Harbor Community Health Centers, Healthcare in Action, Kaiser Permanente, Kedren Community Health Center, Huntington Hospital, Los Angeles Department of Human Services, La Concierge Pharmacy, Long Beach Comprehensive Health Center, Los Angeles Christian Health Center, LGBTQ Center, MedEx Pharmacy, Max Health, Men's Health Foundation, Martin Luther King Jr. Community Hospital, Mend Urgent Care, Mickey Fine Pharmacy, Northeast Valley Health Corporation, Northeast Community Clinic, Mercy Pharmacy, Olympia Plaza Pharmacy, Mental Health America of Los Angeles, Olive

Branch Pharmacy, Passport Health, Planned Parenthood, Paramount Pharmacy, Pico Care Pharmacy, Saban Community Clinic, Albertson-Pavilions Pharmacy, SeraCollection Research Services, St. Anthony Medical Centers, St. John's Community Health, Quiclinics Partners, Tarzana Treatment Centers, Rx Unlimited, St. Anthony Medical Centers, the California Alternate Rates for Energy Program, Southern California Medical Center, University of California at Los Angeles, Venice Family Clinic, University of Southern California (USC) Pharmacy, Via Care Community Health Centers, Visit Healthcare, Watts Healthcare, WesternU Health Pharmacy, the Multi-Service Center the Children's Clinic Family Health, White Memorial Medical Plaza Pharmacy Service, To Help Everyone Health and Wellness Centers, Universal Community Health Center, USC Student Health Keck Medicine, Veritas Testing, Wealth by Health Foundation, Yees Prescription Pharmacy, and CliniCare Pharmacy.

Note. The contents of this article are the responsibility of the authors and do not necessarily represent the official views of nor an endorsement by the CDC, the HHS, or the US government.

CONFLICTS OF INTEREST

The authors have no conflicts of interest to declare.

HUMAN PARTICIPANT PROTECTION

This public health surveillance activity was reviewed and approved by the Los Angeles County Department of Public Health and does not require institutional review board review per the Los Angeles County institutional review board.

REFERENCES

1. County of Los Angeles Public Health. Mpox data. Available at: http://publichealth.lacounty.gov/media/monkeypox/data/index.htm. Accessed July 3, 2023.
2. County of Los Angeles Public Health. Mpox vaccine information. Available at: http://publichealth.lacounty.gov/media/monkeypox/vaccine.htm. Accessed July 3, 2023.
3. County of Los Angeles Public Health. Addressing disproportionality in communities most impacted by mpox. Available at: http://publichealth.lacounty.gov/media/monkeypox/addressing-disproportionality.htm. Accessed December 28, 2022.
4. US Census Bureau. QuickFacts: Los Angeles County, California. Available at: https://www.census.gov/quickfacts/fact/table/losangelescountycalifornia/RHI725221. Accessed June 23, 2023.
5. Centers for Disease Control and Prevention. JYNNEOS vaccine coverage by jurisdiction. August 8, 2023. Available at: https://www.cdc.gov/poxvirus/mpox/cases-data/mpx-jynneos-vaccine-coverage.html. Accessed August 15, 2023.

Reversing Inequity in Mpox Vaccine Distribution, Fulton County, Georgia, June–September 2022

Joshua O'Neal, MA, Jessica Lopes da Rosa, PhD, MPH, Meka Astin, MPH, David Folkes, MD, Dewayne Crowder, and David P. Holland, MD, MHS

Racial/ethnic disparities in the administration of mpox vaccine in Fulton County, Georgia, threatened to undermine the effectiveness of the response. To counteract this inequity, the Fulton County Board of Health partnered with local agencies serving Black and Latino men who have sex with men to coordinate efforts and reserve blocks of time for clients of these agencies to receive a vaccine. The disparities were reversed and approached equity with case rates. (*Am J Public Health*. 2023;113(12):1263–1266. https://doi.org/10.2105/AJPH.2023.307416)

AJPH December 2023, Vol 113, No. 12

On June 17, 2022, the Fulton County Board of Health (FCBOH) began offering expanded postexposure vaccination ("PEP++") for mpox in accordance with guidelines issued by the Centers for Disease Control and Prevention (CDC), although supplies were extremely limited and did not meet the demand. Per guidelines, we offered two doses four weeks apart. Initial events showed large racial/ethnic disparities in vaccine administration favoring White participants, despite the fact that the majority of mpox diagnoses occurred among Black men (Figure 1). To correct these disparities, the FCBOH partnered with community-based organizations (CBOs) serving Black and Latino men who have sex with men to prioritize these constituents.

INTERVENTION AND IMPLEMENTATION

To implement the plan, one day (of three vaccine administration days) per week was reserved for the equity intervention. Each CBO was allocated a number of vaccine appointments on that day based on the size of the CBO and the number of vaccine doses available. The CBOs were responsible for identifying clients meeting vaccine eligibility criteria and notifying them of vaccine availability. Clients were given time periods of availability; strict appointment times were not required. CBOs were also asked to send a representative to the vaccination location to help greet their clients and assist them through the intake process.

Additionally, other measures were taken. Other appointments were released once per week, with an announcement broadcast on social media sites (Instagram, Facebook, Twitter). The time for the release was set at 6 PM to avoid conflict with work hours, and a preannouncement was made earlier in the day when appointments would be released to reduce bias toward those with more access to social media.

PLACE, TIME, AND PERSONS

The intervention included Black and Latino individuals residing in Georgia (not exclusively in Fulton County) meeting the current criteria for expanded postexposure vaccination to mpox (estimated at 27 499). For the majority of the intervention, this included cisgender men or transgender women who had multiple male sexual partners in the preceding 14 days. It also included those with a known exposure to someone diagnosed with mpox.

PEP++ began on June 17, 2022. We concluded the intervention on September 6, 2022, after which time vaccine supply exceeded demand.

PURPOSE

In the first two weeks of vaccine administration, over 70% of the disease burden occurred in non-White persons, whereas over 90% of the vaccines went

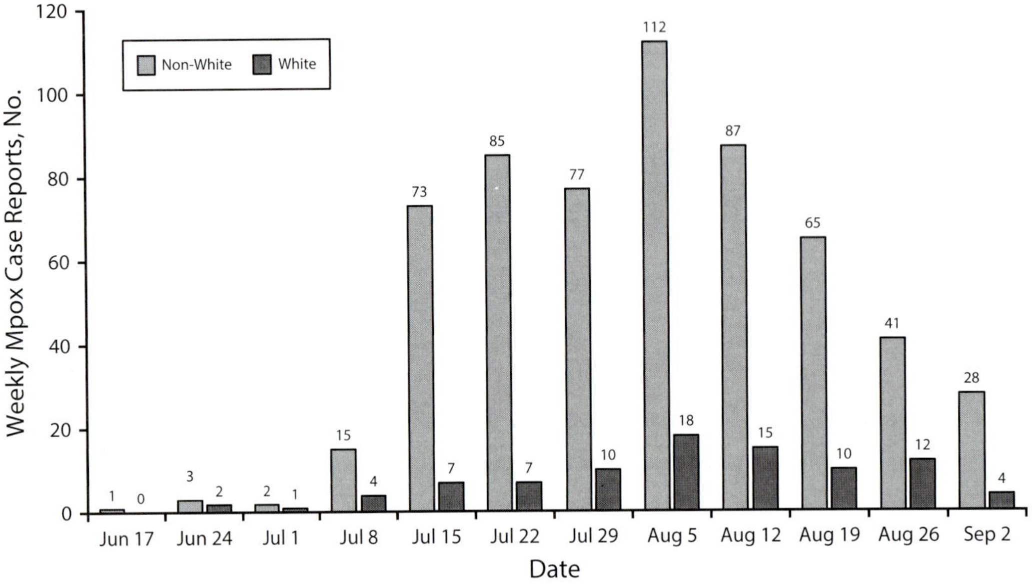

FIGURE 1— Weekly Mpox Case Reports Observed During the Intervention Period: Fulton County, GA, June 17–September 1, 2022

Note. Race for a single individual is unknown and not included.

to White men. The purpose of the intervention was to correct racial/ethnic disparities in vaccine administration and attempt to match vaccine distribution to disease burden.

EVALUATION AND ADVERSE EFFECTS

During the intervention period, a total of 4794 first dose mpox vaccines were administered, with 2851 (59%) given to non-White individuals and 1865 (39%) given to White individuals; 78 (2%) had race unknown. Ninety-nine percent of the recipients were men.

Figure 2 shows the vaccine distribution in two-week intervals and cumulative distribution by race/ethnicity, respectively. A reversal of the disparity occurred by July 26, with a greater number (cumulative) of total vaccines going to Black and Latino recipients by August 2, a trend that was sustained through the end of the intervention.

No serious adverse events occurred as a result of the intervention. However, during the intervention period, the CDC guidelines recommended switching from subcutaneous to intradermal vaccine administration.[1] As a result, many individuals with darker skin experienced hyperpigmentation at the site of intradermal administration, which was considered cosmetically unappealing. In response to feedback from the community, the FCBOH published a fact sheet on hyperpigmentation with guidance on alternative sites of administration (in advance of CDC guidance) and suggestions on minimizing present lesions.[2]

SUSTAINABILITY

Although the formal intervention ended in early September, partnerships with the CBOs to provide mpox vaccinations, primarily through venue-based outreach, continue to the present. The FCBOH plans to expand these partnerships to include support for comprehensive sexual health and health service engagement for persons who use drugs that have been brought into the vaccination clinic.

PUBLIC HEALTH SIGNIFICANCE

Nationwide, mpox disproportionately affected Black and Latino men,[3] whereas vaccines disproportionately went to White men.[4] Imbalances such as this in public health response result in both an ineffective overall response and a worsening of disparities. Recognizing the situation with mpox, the CDC supported two major initiatives for vaccine equity over the Labor Day weekend[5,6] and later launched the Mpox Vaccine Equity Pilot Program.[7] Our equity intervention is the only one that we are aware of that was able to reverse the inequality in vaccine

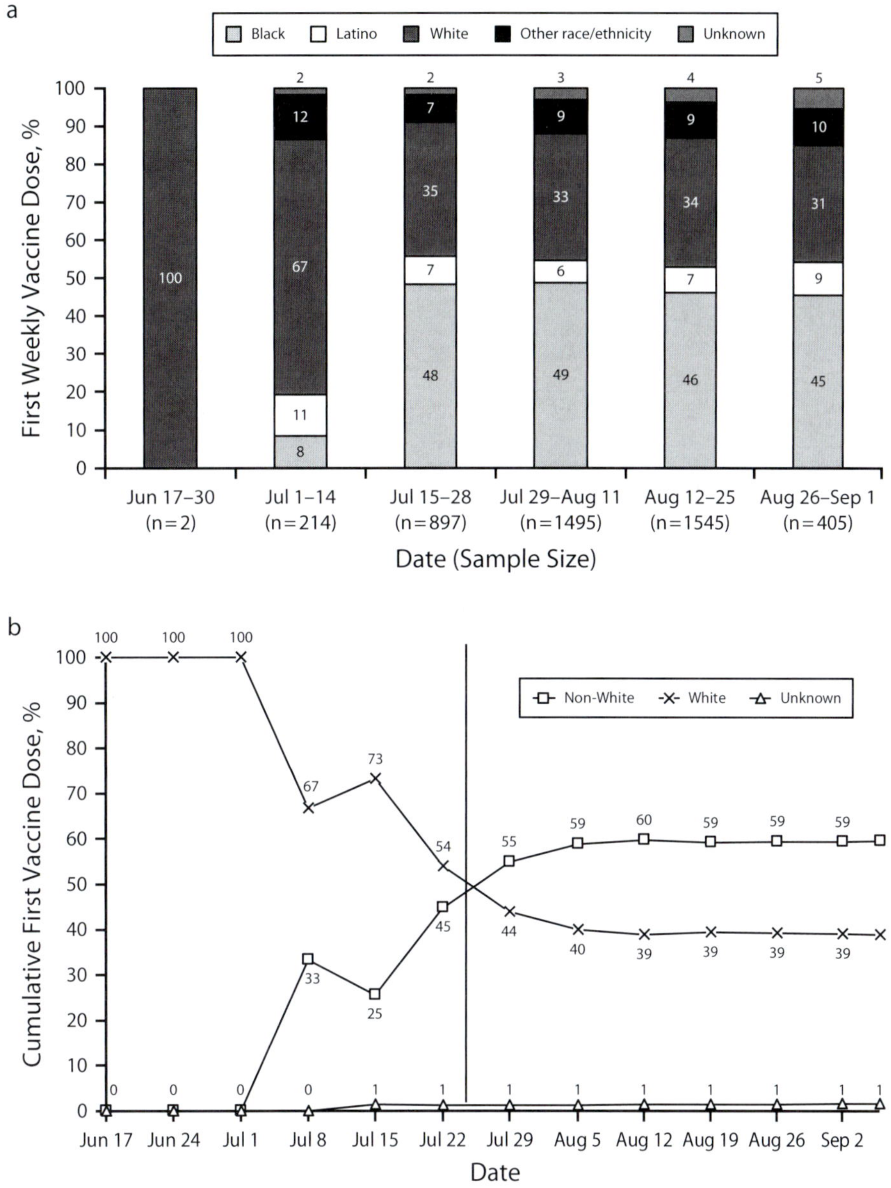

FIGURE 2— Proportion of (a) Vaccine Recipients by 2-Week Interval and Race/Ethnicity, and (b) White vs Non-White Vaccine Recipients Over the Course of the Intervention: Fulton County, GA, June 17–September 6, 2022

Note. Percentages may not add to 100% because of rounding.

distribution early in the epidemic and maintain equity until case rates dropped substantially.

Although our intervention addressed inequities in mpox vaccine distribution, the principles can easily be incorporated into other public health responses. Reserving appointment times and vaccine doses for individuals in the priority populations was the most basic component of the intervention. However, the intervention achieved its success through the close collaboration with organizations serving these disproportionally affected communities. These partnerships enabled messaging to be quickly and accurately disseminated to individuals most likely to benefit from the vaccine. Furthermore, these organizations served as a trusted messenger, which increased the effectiveness of the messaging even further. The communication was two-way, as this channel was the major route by which the FCBOH became aware of the concerns with hyperpigmentation. Such collaborations should be routine across all jurisdictions, as they are essential when addressing concerns in marginalized communities.

During the intervention period, the FCBOH began to add other sexual health services into the vaccine clinic, including HIV testing, preexposure prophylaxis evaluation and initiation, immediate referrals to care for individuals living with HIV but not currently on antiretrovirals, and comprehensive sexually transmitted infection screening. Because these diseases also disproportionately affect Black and Latino men who have sex with men, the vaccine initiative had a secondary effect of increasing sexual health services in these populations. AJPH

ABOUT THE AUTHORS

Joshua O'Neal, Jessica Lopes da Rosa, Meka Astin, and David P. Holland are with the Fulton County Board of Health, Atlanta, GA. David Folkes is with Thrive SS, Atlanta. Dewayne Crowder is with A Vision 4 Hope, Atlanta.

CORRESPONDENCE

Correspondence should be sent to David P. Holland, MD, MHS, FIDSA, 10 Park Place South SE, Atlanta, GA 30303 (e-mail: david.holland@emory.edu). Reprints can be ordered at http://www.ajph.org by clicking the "Reprints" link.

PUBLICATION INFORMATION

Full Citation: O'Neal J, Lopes da Rosa J, Astin M, Folkes D, Crowder D, Holland DP. Reversing inequity in mpox vaccine distribution, Fulton County, Georgia, June–September 2022. *Am J Public Health*. 2023;113(12):1263–1266.

Acceptance Date: August 12, 2023.

DOI: https://doi.org/10.2105/AJPH.2023.307416

CONTRIBUTORS

J. O'Neal and D. P. Holland developed and executed the intervention, and reviewed data and the article. J. Lopes da Rosa analyzed data and reviewed the article. M. Astin, D. Folkes, and D. Crowder executed the intervention and reviewed the article.

CONFLICTS OF INTEREST

The authors have no conflicts of interest to disclose.

HUMAN PARTICIPANT PROTECTION

All data in this analysis were deidentified and therefore exempt from institutional review board review.

REFERENCES

1. Centers for Disease Control and Prevention. JYNNEOS vaccine. Available at: https://www.cdc.gov/poxvirus/monkeypox/interim-considerations/jynneos-vaccine.html. Accessed September 7, 2023.
2. Fulton County Board of Health. Mpox. Available at: https://fultoncountyboh.com/services/epidemiology/mpox. Accessed September 7, 2023.
3. Centers for Disease Control and Prevention. Mpox cases by age and gender, race/ethnicity, and symptoms. Available at: https://www.cdc.gov/poxvirus/monkeypox/response/2022/demographics.html. Accessed January 29, 2023.
4. Centers for Disease Control and Prevention. Mpox vaccine administration in the US. Available at: https://www.cdc.gov/poxvirus/monkeypox/response/2022/vaccines_data.html. Accessed January 29, 2023.
5. Millman AJ, Denson DJ, Allen ML, et al. A health equity approach for implementation of JYNNEOS vaccination at large, community-based LGBTQIA+ events—Georgia, August 27–September 5, 2022. *MMWR Morb Mortal Wkly Rep*. 2022;71(43):1382–1383. https://doi.org/10.15585/mmwr.mm7143e4
6. Soelaeman RH, Mendoza L, McDonald R, et al. Characteristics of JYNNEOS vaccine recipients before and during a large multiday LGBTQIA+ festival—Louisiana, August 9–September 5, 2022. *MMWR Morb Mortal Wkly Rep*. 2022;71(43):1379–1381. https://doi.org/10.15585/mmwr.mm7143e3
7. Centers for Disease Control and Prevention. CDC opening applications for Monkeypox Vaccine Equity Pilot Program. Available at: https://www.cdc.gov/media/releases/2022/p0915-mpx-vaccine-equity.html. Accessed January 29, 2023.

Evaluating e-Connect: Mitigating Race by Gender Disparities in Behavioral Health Referral Among Youths on Probation, Northeast United States, 2019

Margaret E. Ryan, MPH, Katherine S. Elkington, PhD, Casey Sarapas, PhD, Corianna Sichel, PhD, Faye Taxman, PhD, Michael L. Dennis, PhD, and Gail A. Wasserman, PhD

Addressing the behavioral health needs of youths involved in the justice system is key to reducing recidivism risk and preventing long-term system involvement. However, rates of treatment referral and initiation remain low, especially among minoritized youths and boys. The e-Connect System, a digital, clinical decision support system, addresses this problem by increasing rates of behavioral health treatment referral and initiation rates among youths on probation. In this study, we examine whether e-Connect helps improve equity in referral and treatment initiation outcomes. (*Am J Public Health.* 2023;113(12):1267–1270. https://doi.org/10.2105/AJPH.2023.307417)

AJPH December 2023, Vol 113, No. 12

e-Connect, first implemented in 10 county juvenile probation departments in a northeastern state in August 2019, addresses common interagency bridging difficulties between probation and community behavioral health (BH) agencies that contribute to low referral and treatment initiation among youths on probation.

INTERVENTION AND IMPLEMENTATION

e-Connect is a Web-based clinical decision support system, guided by the Gateway Provider Model,[1] designed to help probation officers identify and address youths' BH needs by systematizing evidence-based screening, need identification, referral, and treatment linkage. Compared with baseline (standard probation practice before e-Connect), e-Connect improves BH referral and treatment initiation rates by 11-fold and 16-fold, respectively.[2] However, whether e-Connect addresses or reinforces and exacerbates existing race and gender disparities in these outcomes[3,4] remains unclear. Thus, we examined whether there were disparities in referral and initiation outcomes by race, gender, and their intersection, and if any disparities were reduced during e-Connect. Defining disparities as demographic differences in treatment not justified by the underlying health conditions or treatment preferences,[5] we focused on youths identified with unmet BH treatment need (similar "underlying conditions") and examined BH referral and initiation separately (as the latter might reflect patient preferences, among other factors).

PLACE, TIME, AND PERSONS

We collected administrative records from all new adjusted juvenile delinquent intakes in 10 participating counties from June 1, 2018, through July 31, 2021. Adjusted juvenile delinquents are youths who, following arrest, are assigned to informal probation supervision (as opposed to detention, etc.). This investigation focuses on adjusted juvenile delinquents identified with untreated BH needs via screening at probation intake because it is within probation officers' responsibilities to refer and link them to treatment. Data were split into two comparison groups: baseline (standard probation practice; August 1, 2018–May 31, 2019) and e-Connect (August 1, 2019–July 31, 2021; see Elkington et al.[2] for more details).

e-Connect provides probation officers with automated, standardized, and locally tailored clinical decision support for referring and linking youths to BH treatment. A figure demonstrating the steps of the e-Connect System, including screening, risk classification, referral, and cross-systems linkage, is available online (https://bit.ly/48tqZLQ).

The e-Connect screen measures internalizing disorder, substance use disorder, suicidal thoughts and behaviors, and nonsuicidal self-injury symptoms.[2] The e-Connect System automatically scores youths' responses, assigns them to a suicide risk category (Class I, II, III, and Below Threshold [no BH need]) using an algorithm developed by the research team,[2] and presents the predetermined, county-specific BH referral pathway. Each county's Class I, II, and III referral pathway is developed via an iterative strategic planning process with local probation and BH leadership and details specific referral steps for probation officers to complete.[6] e-Connect generates a referral form summarizing the youth's screening responses and suicide risk level, which the probation officer sends to the designated BH provider. Per the referral pathway, probation officers confirm the youth's treatment attendance with BH.

PURPOSE

Youths in the justice system, most of whom are under community supervision (e.g., probation; 425 000 vs 55 100 in secure care[7]), experience a disproportionately high burden of suicide behaviors and BH needs compared with general population youths.[8] BH treatment helps reduce risk for recidivism and long-term justice involvement.[4,9] Probation officers act as "gatekeepers" to BH care by screening youths for BH need and referring them to community-based treatment services when necessary.[1] However, among probation youths identified with BH need via screening, only one in five are referred to BH and one in 10 initiate treatment.[10] Moreover, minoritized youths and boys in the justice system are historically less likely than others to be referred for care or to initiate care, increasing their risk for long-term justice involvement.[3,4]

Investigators have attributed low referral and treatment initiation rates to probation's unsystematic referral practices and lack of coordination between probation and BH,[10–12] which e-Connect addresses via standardized and coordinated cross-systems referral and linkage procedures. Zeola et al.[4] and Lopez-Willams et al.[3] suggest that consistent, standardized BH referral practices may mitigate treatment disparities related to a youth's race and gender, which we investigate in the present analysis.

EVALUATION AND ADVERSE EFFECTS

We collected records from 405 adjusted juvenile delinquents with untreated BH need (n = 180 baseline, n = 225 e-Connect). The baseline and e-Connect samples were similar in terms of gender (62% and 57% male, respectively), race (58% and 63% White), and offense category (51% and 56% property offense). e-Connect youths were slightly older than baseline youths (mean = 16.51 vs 15.39; $t(404) = -6.7$; $P < .05$), and the distribution of youths per county differed between samples ($\chi^2(2) = 8.8$; $P < .05$).

We used moderated logistic regressions to examine whether there were disparities in rates of BH referral or initiation by race, gender, or their interaction, and whether this changed from baseline to e-Connect implementation, controlling for county, offense category, and age.

Analyses revealed a race by gender by period interaction for BH referral, indicating differential referral practices across race and gender groups during the baseline versus implementation periods (odds ratio [OR] = 21.55; 95% confidence interval [CI] = 1.55, 619.42). Follow-ups within each study period revealed disparities at the intersection of race and gender during the baseline period (race by gender interaction OR = 0.23; 95% CI = 0.06, 0.88). Specifically, planned contrasts showed that non-White girls with identified BH need were less likely to be referred to treatment than White girls (OR = 0.24; 95% CI = 0.06, 0.92), whereas there was no such disparity between non-White and White boys (OR = 1.32; 95% CI = 0.50, 3.47). However, this disparity in referral was mitigated following e-Connect implementation, as neither the race by gender interaction nor main effects for race or gender were significant during the e-Connect period. Table 1 presents rates and relative odds of referral by subgroup.

Among those referred, there were no differences in BH initiation by race and gender, either generally or within either study period. Table 2 presents rates and relative odds of treatment initiation by subgroup.

These results indicate that e-Connect not only improves referral overall but is also associated with improved equity in referral outcomes, supporting the premise that use of consistent, standardized BH referral practices can alleviate treatment disparities among youths in the justice system. The difference in referral at the intersection of race and gender at baseline (non-White girls vs White girls) is especially noteworthy, considering that most research exploring these topics has examined race and gender independently, overlooking the possibility that race- and gender-based inequities may be intersectional rather than merely additive.

TABLE 1— Behavioral Health Referral by Study Period and Demographic Group: Northeast United States, 2019–2021

Subgroup	Period	Race	Gender	No. Referred (%)	Overall OR (95% CI)	Period-Specific OR (95% CI)
Baseline						
White boys	0	0	0	31 (44.3)	1 (Ref)	. . .
White girls	0	0	1	22 (62.9)	2.17 (0.91, 5.36)	. . .
Non-White boys	0	1	0	23 (54.8)	1.76 (0.74, 4.27)	. . .
Non-White girls	0	1	1	12 (36.4)	0.91 (0.34, 2.39)	. . .
e-Connect						
White boys	1	0	0	75 (91.5)	13.50 (5.44, 37.74)	1 (Ref)
White girls	1	0	1	53 (89.8)	11.78 (4.49, 35.64)	1.38 (0.39, 5.19)
Non-White boys	1	1	0	41 (89.1)	14.83 (5.18, 50.37)	2.01 (0.49, 8.90)
Non-White girls	1	1	1	37 (97.4)	66.42 (12.30, 1242.31)	10.73 (1.45, 224.97)

Note. CI = confidence interval; OR = odds ratio. Subgroups are based on (1) period (0 = baseline [i.e., before e-Connect was implemented, when probation departments followed standard practice procedures for identifying behavioral health need and referring and linking youths to care], 1 = e-Connect [i.e., after e-Connect was implemented]); (2) gender (0 = male, 1 = female); and (3) race (0 = White, 1 = non-White). Thus, "Overall OR" represents each subgroup's adjusted odds of receiving a behavioral health referral relative to the odds for White boys during the baseline period. "Period-Specific OR" represents each subgroup's adjusted odds of referral during the e-Connect period relative to the odds for White boys during the e-Connect period. ORs are adjusted for age, county, and offense type.

SUSTAINABILITY

e-Connect is tailored to existing probation and BH system workflows, and it streamlines standard screening, referral, and treatment linkage practices. All 10 sites still use e-Connect, and implementation strategies for scaling up e-Connect are currently being tested in another state.

PUBLIC HEALTH SIGNIFICANCE

We expand prior literature by demonstrating that systematic use of a clinical

TABLE 2— Behavioral Health Initiation by Study Period and Demographic Group: Northeast United States, 2019–2021

Subgroup	Period	Race	Gender	No. Initiated (%)	Overall OR (95% CI)	Period-Specific OR (95% CI)
Baseline						
White boys	0	0	0	11 (35.5)	1 (Ref)	. . .
White girls	0	0	1	7 (31.8)	1.08 (0.31, 3.67)	. . .
Non-White boys	0	1	0	2 (8.7)	0.32 (0.04, 1.53)	. . .
Non-White girls	0	1	1	3 (25.0)	1.71 (0.29, 8.79)	. . .
e-Connect						
White boys	1	0	0	66 (88.0)	17.35 (6.03, 54.94)	1 (Ref)
White girls	1	0	1	46 (86.8)	22.53 (6.96, 83.14)	1.13 (0.38, 3.59)
Non-White boys	1	1	0	31 (75.6)	14.44 (4.56, 50.51)	0.56 (0.17, 1.8)
Non-White girls	1	1	1	32 (86.5)	34.39 (9.08, 154.18)	1.26 (0.32, 5.29)

Note. CI = confidence interval; OR = odds ratio. Subgroups are based on (1) period (0 = baseline [i.e., before e-Connect was implemented, when probation departments followed standard practice procedures for identifying behavioral health need and referring and linking youths to care], 1 = e-Connect [i.e., after e-Connect was implemented]); (2) gender (0 = male, 1 = female); and (3) race (0 = White, 1 = non-White). Thus, "Overall OR" represents each subgroup's adjusted odds of initiating behavioral health treatment relative to the odds for White boys during the baseline period. "Period-Specific OR" represents each subgroup's adjusted odds of treatment initiation during the e-Connect period relative to the odds for White boys during the e-Connect period. ORs are adjusted for age, county, and offense type.

AJPH December 2023, Vol 113, No. 12

decision support system (e-Connect) may mitigate existing race by gender referral disparities in standard probation practice. Considering the elevated suicide risk among youths in the justice system, within the context of the national youth mental health crisis, effective and equitable strategies for linking youths to BH care are critical. Interventions that improve treatment linkage among minoritized youths, who are overrepresented in the juvenile justice system and less likely to make it to care therein, may prevent recidivism[4] and break generational cycles of systemic racism and protracted justice involvement. e-Connect may be useful in other youth-serving settings (e.g., schools, foster care, child welfare) where BH needs are identified in one system and treated in another, necessitating cross-system linkage. Future research should continue to explore the use of e-Connect, and clinical decision support system technology, in facilitating youths' equitable linkage to BH care. AJPH

ABOUT THE AUTHORS

Margaret E. Ryan is with New York State Psychiatric Institute, New York, NY. Katherine S. Elkington, Corianna Sichel, and Gail A. Wasserman are with New York State Psychiatric Institute and Columbia University, New York, NY. Casey Sarapas and Michael L. Dennis are with Chestnut Health Systems, Normal, IL. Faye Taxman is with George Mason University, Fairfax, VA.

CORRESPONDENCE

Correspondence should be sent to Margaret Ryan, 1051 Riverside Dr, New York, NY 10032 (e-mail: margaret.ryan@nyspi.columbia.edu). Reprints can be ordered at http://www.ajph.org by clicking the "Reprints" link.

PUBLICATION INFORMATION

Full Citation: Ryan ME, Elkington KS, Sarapas C, et al. Evaluating e-Connect: mitigating race by gender disparities in behavioral health referral among youths on probation, Northeast United States, 2019. *Am J Public Health*. 2023;113(12): 1267–1270.

Acceptance Date: August 13, 2023.

DOI: https://doi.org/10.2105/AJPH.2023.307417

CONTRIBUTORS

M. E. Ryan led the development of the article, determined the analysis (which was supported by statisticians at Chestnut Health Systems), and led the preparation of literature review, tables, and figures; she is the project director of e-Connect and has worked on the study for over four years. K. S. Elkington and G. A. Wasserman led the research project that this article utilizes data from, advised the development of the article, helped write the article, and provided reviews. C. Sarapas led the statistical analysis and the writing of the results section in the article. C. Sichel helped inform the outline of the article, assisted in writing, and providing review. F. Taxman and M. L. Dennis helped inform the research question, statistical approach, and framing of the research question and findings.

ACKNOWLEDGMENTS

This research is funded by the National Institute of Mental Health (NIMH award 1R01MH11359).

Thank you to two key e-Connect research team members: Alexandra Arnold and Kuljit Dhillon. We are grateful to the probation officers who participated in this work. This work would not have been possible without the partnership and support from our partners within the probation system, both at the state and local level.

Note. The findings and conclusions in this article are those of the authors and do not necessarily represent the official position of the National Institute of Mental Health.

CONFLICTS OF INTEREST

The authors have no conflicts of interest to report.

HUMAN PARTICIPANT PROTECTION

This study was reviewed and approved by the New York State Psychiatric Institute institutional review board (IRB00000488).

REFERENCES

1. Stiffman AR, Pescosolido B, Cabassa LJ. Building a model to understand youth service access: the gateway provider model. *Ment Health Serv Res.* 2004;6(4):189–198. https://doi.org/10.1023/B:MHSR.0000044745.09952.33
2. Elkington KS, Wasserman GA, Ryan ME, et al. e-Connect: linking probation youth at risk for suicide to behavioral health services. *J Consult Clin Psychol.* 2023;91(9):547–557. https://psycnet.apa.org/doi/10.1037/ccp0000824
3. Lopez-Williams A, Stoep AV, Kuo E, Stewart DG. Predictors of mental health service enrollment among juvenile offenders. *Youth Violence Juv Justice.* 2006;4(3):266–280. https://doi.org/10.1177/1541204006290159
4. Zeola MP, Guina J, Nahhas RW. Mental health referrals reduce recidivism in first-time juvenile offenders, but how do we determine who is referred? *Psychiatr Q.* 2017;88(1):167–183. https://doi.org/10.1007/s11126-016-9445-z
5. Institute of Medicine. *Unequal Treatment: Confronting Racial and Ethnic Disparities in Health Care.* Washington, DC: National Academies Press; 2003.
6. Wasserman GA, Elkington KS, Robson G, Taxman F. Bridging juvenile justice and behavioral health systems: development of a clinical pathways approach to connect youth at risk for suicidal behavior to care. *Health Justice.* 2021;9(1):36. https://doi.org/10.1186/s40352-021-00164-4
7. Hockenberry S, Puzzanchera C. *Juvenile Court Statistics 2019.* Pittsburgh, PA: National Center for Juvenile Justice; 2021.
8. Wasserman GA, McReynolds LS, Schwalbe CS, Keating JM, Jones SA. Psychiatric disorder, comorbidity, and suicidal behavior in juvenile justice youth. *Crim Justice Behav.* 2010;37(12):1361–1376. https://doi.org/10.1177/0093854810382751
9. Hoeve M, McReynolds LS, Wasserman GA. The influence of adolescent psychiatric disorder on young adult recidivism. *Crim Justice Behav.* 2013;40(12):1368–1382. https://doi.org/10.1177/0093854813488106
10. Wasserman GA, McReynolds LS, Taxman FS, et al. The missing link(age): multilevel contributors to service uptake failure among youths on community justice supervision. *Psychiatr Serv.* 2021;72(5):546–554. https://doi.org/10.1176/appi.ps.202000163
11. Dennis ML, Smith CN, Belenko S, et al. Operationalizing a behavioral health services cascade of care model: lessons learned from a 33-site implementation in juvenile justice community supervision. *Fed Probat.* 2019;83(2):52–64. Available at: https://www.ncbi.nlm.nih.gov/pmc/articles/PMC8341285/. Accessed December 10, 2022.
12. Elkington KS, Lee J, Brooks C, Watkins J, Wasserman GA. Falling between two systems of care: engaging families, behavioral health and the justice systems to increase uptake of substance use treatment in youth on probation [erratum in *J Subst Abuse Treat.* 2020;114:108010]. *J Subst Abuse Treat.* 2020;112:49–59. https://doi.org/10.1016/j.jsat.2020.01.008

Child Safety Seat–Use Behavior Among Parents of Newborns: A Trans-Theoretical Model–Guided Intervention in Shantou, China, 2021

Yixiang Peng, MD, Feng Wu, MD, Jingzhen Yang, PhD, and Liping Li, PhD

We evaluated the effect of a trans-theoretical model–based intervention on child safety seat (CSS)–use behaviors among parents of newborns in Shantou, China. Parents' knowledge, attitude, and self-efficacy scores on CSS use were significantly higher at one, three, and six months after the intervention compared with scores at baseline. Parents' stage of CSS use also advanced as the intervention progressed. The trans-theoretical model–based intervention and evidence generated from this study may provide guidance for future individualized interventions to improve CSS use. (*Am J Public Health*. 2023;113(12):1271–1275. https://doi.org/10.2105/AJPH.2023.307415)

AJPH December 2023, Vol 113, No. 12

In China, more than 20 000 children are killed or injured in motor vehicle crashes (MVCs) each year, with more than one third occurring during car rides.[1] Child safety seat (CSS) use can reduce the risk of MVC-related injury by 71% to 82%, and MVC-related death by 28%.[2,3] However, the rate of CSS use in China is only about 20%, considerably lower than that in other developed countries.[4,5] Implementing effective intervention strategies is urgently needed to increase CSS use. Furthermore, previous interventions promoting CSS use often applied "one-size-fits-all" strategies without accounting for motivational and individual differences.[6,7]

The trans-theoretical model (TTM) emphasizes the importance of understanding each individual's needs, intentions, and readiness for behavior change, as well as the respective stage of behavior change that each individual is in before implementing individualized, targeted interventions to produce a series of continuous and progressive behavior changes.[8] To date, TTM-based interventions have been widely used to promote health behaviors, including physical activity and chronic disease management, and have allowed greater sensitivity in measuring behavior change progression than traditional interventions.[9,10] Thus, TTM-based interventions may help to improve CSS use among parents of newborns.

INTERVENTION AND IMPLEMENTATION

We designed and implemented a TTM-based intervention that targeted parents of newborns ("parents"), aiming to advance parents' stage of change regarding CSS use and, ultimately, to increase the use of CSSs. We used a pre- and posttest study design. We provided a baseline survey to each parent following their written informed consent that included a question to assess the stage of change in CSS-use behavior (Table A, available as a supplement to the online version of this article at https://ajph.org). We then implemented the intervention components of motivational interviewing tailored to one of five stages of change that parents were in (Table 1).

All parents participated in both an onsite intervention and an online intervention via WeChat that lasted six months. However, the intervention was delivered with different strategies, content focus, and frequency based on parents' stage of change in CSS-use behavior (Table 1). We collected study outcome data at baseline as well as at one, three, and six months after the intervention by phone, WeChat, or online survey. We used 41 questions to collect data on demographics, stage of change, knowledge, attitudes, self-efficacy, and behaviors regarding CSS

TABLE 1— Program Characteristics, Interview Content, and Strategies for Changing Child Safety Seat (CSS)–Use Behavior in Each Stage of Change: Shantou, China, 2021

Stages of Change	Characteristics	Interview Content	Strategies
Precontemplation[a]	Not considering the use of CSS	Relevance	Understand reasons for parents' reluctance to use CSSs and their feelings and opinions on using CSSs. Introduce and describe some cases of road traffic accidents involving children. Guide the parents to recall their own car riding experience. Provide information on the current situation of child road traffic injuries and misconceptions about riding.
Contemplation[a]	Beginning to consider using CSS but do not want to take action yet and have no clear plan	Risk	Identify the complex psychology of parents who plan to use CSSs but are reluctant to take some immediate actions. Analyze the impact of rides without CSSs on child passengers and how CSSs protect child passengers. Introduce CSS types and options. Provide information on case studies of children's road traffic accidents and proper car riding practices.
Preparation[a]	Intending to take action to make changes and to start building a usage plan	Reward	Understand CSS-use plans made by parents. Identify the problems and obstacles that can occur in CSS-use behavioral change. Provide alternative solutions and techniques. Provide information about the benefits of using CSSs and the risks of nonuse. Guide parents to make a public commitment to using CSSs regularly.
Action[b]	Have started using CSS regularly but for ≤6 mo	Roadblock	Recognize and encourage the use of CSSs. Provide materials such as posters related to the proper use of CSS. Encourage parents to insist on using the CSS even if their child refuses or find it troublesome to install and dismantle, rather than complete nonuse. Uncover the reasons why parents who have tried to use CSSs before could not persist. Assess the detrimental factors that impede CSS-use behaviors and discuss strategies to address these issues.
Maintenance[c]	Have been using CSS for >6 mo, with relatively stable behavior	Repetition	Give parents positive affirmation to use CSSs regularly and encourage them to persist. Strengthen the links among CSS use and child passenger safety (e.g., reducing head impacts, supporting the baby's body and spine).

Note. The duration of onsite and WeChat interventions was 6 months. The WeChat intervention was implemented one or two times per week at each stage of change.
[a]The onsite intervention occurred once for 10 to 15 minutes per person.
[b]The onsite intervention occurred once every two weeks for 10 to 15 minutes per person.
[c]The onsite intervention occurred once per month for 10 to 15 minutes per person.

use (Tables A to E, available as supplements to the online version of this article at https://ajph.org). The content of the questionnaire was the same at baseline and at follow-ups, and it took parents 15 to 20 minutes to complete.

We used SPSS 21.0 (IBM, Somers, NY) to carry out statistical analyses. We used a repeated measures one-way analysis of variance to compare continuous outcome data before and after the intervention, followed by the Bonferroni posttest. We used the χ^2 test for trends to compare count data before and after the intervention.

PLACE, TIME, AND PERSONS

The study included parents in five randomly selected confinement centers (postnatal rehabilitation institutions that provide postnatal care, postnatal recovery, and health training for mothers and their babies who have just been discharged from hospital) located in Shantou, China. The program was implemented from April 1 to November 31, 2021. We assessed and analyzed the stages of change in CSS use after a baseline survey (April–June 2021) and then implemented a TTM-based intervention. Parents were eligible if they

1. were parents of newborns,
2. had no serious postpartum complications for the newborn or mother,
3. owned a private car,
4. had WeChat, and
5. agreed to participate in the study through signed consent.

All participants completed the study voluntarily and were not compensated.

PURPOSE

CSS use has been proven to be the most effective tool for protecting child occupants in MVCs. However, compared with developed countries, CSS use is considerably lower in China. The aim of this study was to evaluate a TTM-based intervention approach for improvement of knowledge and behaviors of CSS use among parents of newborns.

EVALUATION AND ADVERSE EFFECTS

A total of 180 parents were eligible and enrolled in the study; 27 were lost to follow-up after six months of the intervention. There was no difference between study participants and dropouts at baseline. The demographic characteristics of participating parents and children are shown in Table F (available as a supplement to the online version of this article at https://ajph.org). Of 180 parents enrolled, 51.7% were female, and 43.3% were aged 26 to 30 years. The distribution of the stages of change in parents before the intervention was 54.4%, 22.8%, 11.1%, 6.7%, and 5.0% in precontemplation, contemplation, preparation, action, and maintenance stages, respectively.

Improving Knowledge and Practice

Parents' knowledge, attitudes, and self-efficacy scores were significantly higher after the intervention compared with scores at baseline (Table 2). Parents' knowledge score, attitudes score, and general self-efficacy score at six months after the intervention was 3.07 (95% confidence interval [CI] = 2.85, 3.29), 7.24 (95% CI = 6.41, 8.08), and 5.78 (95% CI = 4.68, 6.88) points higher than that at baseline, respectively (Table G, available as a supplement to the online version of this article at https://ajph.org). Moreover, parents showed greater improvement in behavior after TTM-based intervention, especially in purchase of CSS and CSS-use behavior (frequency, installation location, orientation, whether it is checked before use and after children are put into it and the seat belt is fastened). Compared with baseline, the purchase rate of CSS increased six months after the intervention (47.7% vs 26.8%; $P = .001$). The percentage of parents who always used CSS increased (28.8% vs 14.6%; $P = .038$). Among parents who used CSS, more parents installed CSS in the back row middle position (46.3% vs 4.8%; $P = .011$), used backward-facing installation (48.1% vs 19.0%; $P = .036$), and checked the CSS before use (66.7% vs 28.6%; $P = .011$) six months after the intervention compared with their baseline before the intervention.

Advancing Stage of Change

The distribution of stages of change in parents at one month following the intervention was not significantly different from that at baseline ($\chi^2 = 4.199$; $P = .380$). However, as the intervention proceeded, the stages of change showed a trend toward advanced stages ($\chi^2 = 33.246$; $P < .001$). Compared with the baseline stages of change, the stage span of CSS use among parents increased as the intervention progressed.

SUSTAINABILITY

The lack of national legislation mandating CSS use, coupled with low parental awareness and misconceptions about child passenger safety, may have contributed to the considerably low CSS usage in China. In this study, the TTM-based intervention utilized five different approaches appropriate to parents in each of five stages of change, which were shown to significantly improve parents' CSS-use behaviors. Moreover, in this study, we made a guideline poster on the implementation of interventions based on the TTM and explained it to the researchers, which facilitated the formation and continuity of best practices for increasing CSS use. Given participants in this study were not evenly distributed across the five stages of change, future studies should explore effective strategies that target specific stage(s) of change for improving CSS use.

PUBLIC HEALTH SIGNIFICANCE

To the best of our knowledge, this study is the first to apply a TTM-based intervention to improve the CSS-use behavior of parents of newborns. To better understand the context of this study, it is important to note that TTM divides individual behavior change into five stages of change, and each stage corresponds to different readiness and intention to change a behavior,

AJPH December 2023, Vol 113, No. 12

TABLE 2— Comparative Analysis of Knowledge, Attitudes, and Self-Efficacy Scores and Child Safety Seat (CSS)–Related Situations of Parents: Shantou, China, 2021

	Intervention Time Points, Mean ± SD or No. (%)					
Items	T_0	T_1	T_3	T_6	F or χ^2	*P*
Knowledge scores	2.60 ± 0.83	3.75 ± 0.89	5.04 ± 0.97	5.67 ± 0.79	576.983	< .001
Attitudes scores	19.05 ± 3.35	22.30 ± 2.58	25.36 ± 3.42	26.29 ± 3.18	336.338	< .001
General self-efficacy scores	21.49 ± 3.36	23.78 ± 2.10	25.95 ± 3.70	27.27 ± 5.08	127.459	< .001
Purchased CSS					14.384	.001
Yes	41 (26.8)		60 (39.2)	73 (47.7)		
No	112 (73.2)		93 (60.8)	80 (52.3)		
Frequency of CSS use[a]					16.324	.038[b]
Always	6 (14.6)		11 (18.3)	21 (28.8)		
Often	11 (26.8)		24 (40.0)	25 (34.2)		
Sometimes	2 (4.9)		7 (11.7)	8 (11.0)		
Seldom	2 (4.9)		0	0		
Never	20 (48.8)		18 (30.0)	19 (26.0)		
Installation location in back row					13.020	.011
Left	12 (57.1)		16 (37.2)	17 (31.5)		
Middle	1 (4.8)		12 (27.9)	25 (46.3)		
Right	8 (38.1)		15 (34.9)	12 (22.2)		
Installation orientation					6.654	.036
Forward	17 (81.0)		31 (72.1)	28 (51.9)		
Backward	4 (19.0)		12 (27.9)	26 (48.1)		
Whether CSS is checked before use and after children are put into CSS					8.939	.011
Yes	6 (28.6)		23 (53.5)	36 (66.7)		
No	15 (71.4)		20 (46.5)	18 (33.3)		

Note. The sample size was n = 153.
[a]Take 10 travels as a unit: always ≥ 9 times; often = 6–8 times; sometimes = 3–5 times; seldom = 1 or 2 times.
[b]Based on Fisher exact test.

providing effective guidance for changing individual behavior. This study provides in-depth and new insights for interventions aimed at improving the use of CSS. The TTM-based intervention, which demonstrated improved knowledge and increased CSS use in the current study, could be further applied to promote the use of CSS. AJPH

ABOUT THE AUTHORS

Yixiang Peng, Feng Wu, and Liping Li are with the School of Public Health, Shantou University, and Injury Prevention Research Center, Shantou University Medical College, Shantou, China. Y. Peng is also with the Department of Prevention and Healthcare and Healthcare-Associated Infection Management, The Third People's Hospital of Shenzhen, Shenzhen, China. Jingzhen Yang is with the Center for Injury Research and Policy, Abigail Wexner Research Institute at Nationwide Children's Hospital, Columbus, OH.

CORRESPONDENCE

Correspondence should be sent to Liping Li, Daxue Road 243, Shantou City, Guangdong, China (e-mail: lpli@stu.edu.cn). Reprints can be ordered at https://ajph.org by clicking the "Reprints" link.

PUBLICATION INFORMATION

Full Citation: Peng Y, Wu F, Yang J, Li L. Child safety seat–use behavior among parents of newborns: a trans-theoretical model–guided intervention in Shantou, China, 2021. *Am J Public Health*. 2023; 113(12):1271–1275.

Acceptance Date: August 14, 2023.

DOI: https://doi.org/10.2105/AJPH.2023.307415

CONTRIBUTORS

L. Li conceptualized and designed the study. Y. Peng collected, cleaned, and analyzed the data and wrote the original article. F. Wu revised and edited the article. J. Yang supervised, revised, and edited the article.

ACKNOWLEDGMENTS

Funding for this work has been provided by the Shantou Health Care Category Science and Technology Project (grant STYL2022015).

All authors acknowledge the selected participants and all survey staff for their support.

Note. The funding agency had no role in study design, data collection, analysis or interpretation of data, writing the manuscript, and decision to submit the article for publication.

CONFLICTS OF INTEREST

The authors have no conflicts of interest to declare.

HUMAN PARTICIPANT PROTECTION

This study was conducted strictly based on the Declaration of Helsinki and approved by the Ethics Committee of the Shantou University Medical College (No. SUMC-2021-86).

REFERENCES

1. China Center for Disease Control and Prevention, China Chronic Noncommunicable Disease Control and Prevention Center, Statistical Information Center of the National Health and Family Planning Commission. China death cause monitoring data set 2017[M]. Beijing, China: Science and Technology of China Press; 2018
2. Sauber-Schatz EK, West BA, Bergen G; Centers for Disease Control and Prevention. Vital signs: restraint use and motor vehicle occupant death rates among children aged 0–12 years—United States, 2002–2011. *MMWR Morb Mortal Wkly Rep.* 2014;63(5):113–118. Available at: https://www.cdc.gov/mmwr/preview/mmwrhtml/mm6305a8.htm. Accessed May 27, 2023.
3. Durbin DR; Committee on Injury, Violence, and Poison Prevention. Child passenger safety. *Pediatrics.* 2011;127(4):788–793. https://doi.org/10.1542/peds.2011-0213
4. Zheng X, Li R, Yang H, et al. The rate of child restraint system use among children aged under six years in China. *Scand J Public Health.* 2022;50(8):1192–1198. https://doi.org/10.1177/14034948211036621
5. Cai W, Lei L, Zhou H, et al. Child restraint system use and its associated factors in Shenzhen. *Accid Anal Prev.* 2021;160:106321. https://doi.org/10.1016/j.aap.2021.106321
6. Lei H, Gao R, Yang J, Li L. Parent-based intervention to improve child restraint use among kindergarteners in China. *Am J Public Health.* 2018;108(11):1524–1526. https://doi.org/10.2105/AJPH.2018.304650
7. Keay L, Hunter K, Brown J, et al. Evaluation of an education, restraint distribution, and fitting program to promote correct use of age-appropriate child restraints for children aged 3 to 5 years: a cluster randomized trial. *Am J Public Health.* 2012;102(12):e96–e102. https://doi.org/10.2105/AJPH.2012.301030
8. Prochaska JO, Velicer WF. The transtheoretical model of health behavior change. *Am J Health Promot.* 1997;12(1):38–48. https://doi.org/10.4278/0890-1171-12.1.38
9. Adams J, White M. Are activity promotion interventions based on the transtheoretical model effective? A critical review. *Br J Sports Med.* 2003;37(2):106–114. https://doi.org/10.1136/bjsm.37.2.106
10. Winter SJ, Sheats JL, King AC. The use of behavior change techniques and theory in technologies for cardiovascular disease prevention and treatment in adults: a comprehensive review. *Prog Cardiovasc Dis.* 2016;58(6):605–612. https://doi.org/10.1016/j.pcad.2016.02.005

Toward More Equitable Public Health Data: An *AJPH* Special Section

Ninez A. Ponce, PhD, MPP, and Denys T. Lau, PhD

ABOUT THE AUTHORS

Ninez A. Ponce is with the Fielding School of Public Health, University of California, Los Angeles. Denys T. Lau was an AJPH *associate editor and is with the Bloomberg School of Public Health, Johns Hopkins University, Baltimore, MD.*

See also Toward More Equitable Public Health Data, pp. 1278–1308.

The renewed attention to health equity highlights the importance of ensuring that everyone, regardless of their social position, resources, or circumstances, can attain optimal health. To achieve health equity, high-quality equity research is needed to produce evidence for effective policy and programmatic decision-making. Much has been written about how health research can be conducted more equitably. For instance, to be equitable, research should reject the notion that research can be culture free,[1] should require that researchers have a deep understanding of the history and consequences of power and racism in their fields,[2] and should account for the differences in biases and assumptions between researchers as the standard position and communities as mere participants.[3]

To support equitable research, public health data need to be more equitable, but the topic of equitable public health data has received less attention. Transforming public health data systems to become more equity centered is the focus of a recent Robert Wood Johnson National Commission to Transform Public Health Data Systems Foundation report titled "Charting a Course for an Equity-Centered Data System."[4] The commission presents recommendations on what is needed to transform the data narrative (i.e., a way of seeing the world that can reinforce social norms and expectations) in the United States.

Public health data are frequently used to track community problems and rationalize investments after the fact, sometimes to the detriment of historically underrepresented and marginalized communities. To transform this data narrative, key sectors must ensure that the current elements of data (e.g., measures and indicators) do not perpetuate systemic inequities. If public health data systems cannot collect more precise demographic measures of race and ethnicity, disability status, sexual orientation and gender identity, and language-bridging needs effectively, it becomes difficult to address health equity. At the heart of the commission's message of transformation is the need to develop governance structures that value equity, use the diversity of data across sectors, and include new principles of data stewardship.

This special section of *AJPH* furthers the discourse on how we can build more equitable public health data and data systems. The approaches entail creating better data content, processes, and infrastructures. Public health data should include elements for identifying health inequities and tracking our progress toward greater health equity locally and nationally. There needs to be more standardized data on structural and perceived racism and other forms of discrimination and exclusion using validated measures, more representative data with sufficient sample sizes to disaggregate and identify the experiences and needs of marginalized communities, and more ongoing data collection to monitor progress toward health equity.

Additionally, the processes by which public health data are collected, analyzed, disseminated, and translated need to be equitable, diverse, inclusive, and accessible. For instance, there needs to be more effective approaches using data across multiple sectors and disciplines beyond public health and medicine, greater data transparency and broader public data accessibility, and more meaningful community engagement that does not overburden disadvantaged communities.

Finally, public health data that are stored and maintained should be usable by, viable for, and trustworthy to all people. There needs to be greater data standards and interoperability across different systems, more funding and resource opportunities to sustain these systems, and greater data security and privacy to reduce disclosure risk and potential harm to communities. The articles in this special section provide insights and examples from federal, state, and local perspectives and experiences on how our nation's public health survey and surveillance programs can become more equitable.

O'Hara and Rhodes (p. 1278) share examples of how federal agencies are building capacity to produce equitable data, such as requiring data definitions to reflect changes in our society, changing practices that historically have disadvantaged certain groups, and investing in new methods and technologies to use population data sets.

Sheingold et al. (p. 1301) propose a framework on upstream structural factors and downstream consequences associated with the distribution of social determinants of health and discuss the public health data needed to evaluate federal policies and their progress toward health equity under the framework.

Sharma et al. (p. 1283) discuss how California is advancing infrastructure to support data sharing and data analytics between the state's Medicaid and public health programs to understand and manage the health of specific populations, address racial/ethnic biases in public health data, and advance health equity.

Gundanna et al. (p. 1296) describe their advocacy work involving community building and budget allocations to champion the first-ever data disaggregation law for Asian Americans, Native Hawaiians, and Pacific Islanders in New York City and State.

Baker et al. (p. 1287) discuss the barriers to interoperability and use of sexual orientation and gender identity data in electronic health records across health care institutions, which limit the ability to support evidence-based interventions and further sexual and minority population health improvement.

These articles provide proof of concept for equity-centered data across diverse sectors and perspectives. We hope this special section inspires action and spurs progress toward achieving more equitable public health data systems. Furthermore, this special section follows two previously published special sections in *AJPH* building on the central theme of establishing more accurate, reliable, equitable, and resilient surveillance and survey data systems in the wake of the COVID-19 pandemic: reinventing and reestablishing public health surveillance and survey programs in the United States (https://ajph.aphapublications.org/toc/ajph/111/12) and addressing public health data gaps to better understand, track, and reduce the disparate effects of COVID-19 among disadvantaged populations (https://ajph.aphapublications.org/toc/ajph/112/10). AJPH

CORRESPONDENCE

Correspondence should be sent to Denys T. Lau, PhD, Department of Health Policy and Management, 624 N Broadway, Baltimore, MD 21205 (e-mail: dlau1@jhu.edu). Reprints can be ordered at http://www.ajph.org by clicking the "Reprints" link.

PUBLICATION INFORMATION

Full Citation: Ponce NA, Lau DT. Toward more equitable public health data: an *AJPH* special section. *Am J Public Health*. 2023;113(12):1276–1277.

Acceptance Date: September 17, 2023.

DOI: https://doi.org/10.2105/AJPH.2023.307468

CONTRIBUTORS

Both authors drafted, revised, and approved the editorial.

CONFLICTS OF INTEREST

We have no potential or actual conflicts of interest from funding or affiliation-related activities to disclose.

REFERENCES

1. Westat JF, Frierson H, Katzenmeyer C; National Science Foundation. *The 2002 User-Friendly Handbook for Project Evaluation*. January 2002. Available at: https://www.nsf.gov/pubs/2002/nsf02057/nsf02057.pdf. Accessed September 12, 2023.
2. Farrell L. Equitable research requires questioning the status quo. September 20, 2021. Available at: https://www.urban.org/urban-wire/equitable-research-requires-questioning-status-quo. Accessed September 12, 2023.
3. Annie E. Casey Foundation. Step-by-step guide on using equity principles in social science research. October 6, 2019. Available at: https://www.aecf.org/blog/step-by-step-guide-on-using-equity-principles-in-social-science-research. Accessed September 12, 2023.
4. Robert Wood Johnson Foundation, National Commission to Transform Public Health Data Systems. Charting a course for an equity-centered data system. October 1, 2021. Available at: https://www.rwjf.org/en/insights/our-research/2021/10/charting-a-course-for-an-equity-centered-data-system.html. Accessed September 12, 2023.

The Federal Agencies' Hidden Efforts to Produce Equitable Data

Amy O'Hara, PhD, and Rosemary Rhodes, BA

ABOUT THE AUTHORS

Amy O'Hara and Rosemary Rhodes are with the Massive Data Institute at the McCourt School of Public Policy, Georgetown University, Washington, DC.

See also Toward More Equitable Public Health Data, pp. 1276–1308.

The COVID-19 pandemic illustrated the US government's inability to effectively respond to a public health emergency in a timely manner. Data quality and availability issues hindered efforts to understand disparities in health outcomes, such as the disproportionate impact of the pandemic on Black and Latino populations. Despite the Centers for Disease Control and Prevention's temporary authorization to gather and share data, inadequate capacity and infrastructure resulted in delayed detection and response, which cost millions of American lives.

The public health data ecosystem lacked methods to normalize and synthesize information from thousands of outdated systems and standards to aid in that normalization. Legal, political, and cultural barriers prevented information sharing. However, efforts to address these obstacles are underway, with multiple agencies working to remedy the lack of relevant and timely data for all socio-demographic groups. We highlight a selection of federal initiatives that are investing in equitable data.

IMPROVING DEMOGRAPHIC DATA

Many federal agencies are actively working on equity issues and complying with executive orders[1,2] to advance racial equity and support for underserved communities. This section focuses on federal initiatives involving data collection, particularly activities in the US Department of Health and Human Services (HHS), Census Bureau, and Office of Management and Budget (OMB) to improve demographic data collection and standardization.

Through the Equitable Data Working Group,[3] chaired by the OMB, agencies are improving methods to collect data that can be disaggregated across population groups and relevant geographies. For the first time since 1997, OMB plans to revise Statistical Policy Directive No. 15: Standards for Maintaining, Collecting, and Presenting Federal Data on Race and Ethnicity to ensure that federal agencies are collecting comparable, representative data. As OMB notes, there have been "large societal, political, economic, and demographic shifts in the United States" during the last 25 years, necessitating a review of the standards[4] to reflect increased racial and ethnic diversity in the United States and to accurately depict growing numbers of people who identify as more than one racial or ethnic category.

The Census Bureau has collected data on race since the first census in 1790 and on Hispanic or Latino origin since 1970. The Census Bureau regularly assesses the quality and completeness of its data. Nine million people reported multiple race groups in 2010; that number rose to 33.8 million in 2020. Under the current standards, race is collected separately from ethnicity. Research indicates that a growing number of Hispanic respondents are not selecting a race or choosing "Some Other Race." This was confirmed in the 2020 Census, when nearly 50 million people identified as "Some Other Race" (45.3 million people of Hispanic or Latino origin were classified as "Some Other Race" either alone or in combination, compared with only 4.6 million people who were not of Hispanic or Latino origin). Census Bureau research has demonstrated that more specific and accurate responses are obtained when using a "combined question" that asks what categories describe a person. Such question changes can ensure that our increasingly diverse population is accurately reflected in data.

Statistical Policy Directive No. 15 review is also considering adding a new minimum race category for Middle Eastern or North African (MENA). Adding a MENA race category[5] will give people descending from 22 Arab countries, three non-Arab MENA countries, and three transnational communities visibility in data. MENA data could then be used in health and social science research, including research to improve immigrant and language services, and hate crime reporting.

Administrative data and electronic health records also have data collection problems for race and ethnicity. In the public health sphere, 70% of fields for race and ethnicity are missing on electronic health records.[6] State data systems are missing race and ethnicity data for large fractions of their client

AJPH December 2023, Vol 113, No. 12

records as well. For example, data on race and ethnicity are regularly missing in state eligibility and claims systems, limiting the Centers for Medicare and Medicaid Services' (CMS's) ability to assess program utilization and characteristics of Medicaid enrollees. A recent Census Bureau study found that 19% of Medicaid beneficiaries were missing race data overall, but the missingness varied widely by states. This report, "Enhancing Race and Ethnicity Information in Medicaid Data,"[7] illustrated how decennial census and American Community Survey data can fill in the missing information to produce statistics, reducing the percentage with missing information from 19% to 7%. Such efforts will address a growing data gap: a 2022 CMS report noted that in 2016, seven states reported missing race/ethnicity information for 50% or more of their beneficiaries.

Neglecting to correctly measure and capture an increasingly diverse population undermines ongoing federal efforts to achieve health equity. For example, a recent Kaiser Family Foundation study[8] found that when Asian subcategories are aggregated, the population may appear to fare better than White populations across various indicators. The report highlights the variation in the uninsured rate between Asian and Native Hawaiian and other Pacific Islander (NHOPI) subgroups, finding that NHOPI subgroups are more likely to be uninsured compared with the Asian population—a finding that is lost when the Asian subcategories are combined. Broad racial aggregation can also distort other variations in economic and health outcomes, which can lead to federal programs and policies inadvertently misallocating investment into less needy groups.

Improvements to demographic data extend beyond race and ethnicity, with important work underway regarding sexual orientation and gender identity (SOGI). Building on a decade of work across federal agencies,[9] best practices[10] have emerged to capture data beyond male and female designations. SOGI research and testing are underway on various data collections across agencies. The Collaborating Center for Questionnaire Design and Evaluation Research at the National Center for Health Statistics (NCHS) is currently leading efforts to design, test, and implement various SOGI questions for federal surveys and other government agency data collections, such as a single, nonbinary gender question for federal health surveys.[11] Collecting SOGI will enable research on health disparities suffered by lesbian, gay, bisexual, transgender, queer or questioning, intersex, and asexual individuals, such as differential cancer rates and risks of anxiety and depression.

Beyond these efforts to improve demographic data collections, efforts are also underway to improve other data elements sought by equity assessments. The Census Bureau is blending data from surveys, censuses, and administrative records to improve data on earnings, addressing missingness and underreporting by using multiple sources of data, illustrated in the National Experimental Wellbeing Statistics[12] project. More accurate income data will lead to better studies of inequality and economic mobility. The Census Bureau is exploring methods to measure citizenship using administrative data,[13] a worthy (and politically charged) project since self-response rates on that variable have dropped steadily in the American Community Survey.[14]

These efforts are likely to transform how we measure our population. The Equitable Data Working Group recommended capacity building to assess equity within and across data sources.[15] Researchers should encourage transparency in these assessments and ensure that agencies consider how data collections impact measures of disparities and outcomes and support resources across agencies to maintain complete, comparable data.

IMPROVING EQUITABLE ACCESS TO DATA

Data access has not been equitable; in too many cases, access relied on personal connections and unwritten rules. Federal agencies have publicized their data inventories and learning agendas as directed by the Foundations for Evidence-Based Policymaking Act[16] (the "Evidence Act"). The Evidence Act requires agencies to name a chief data officer, evaluation officer, and statistical official to improve the collection, management, analysis, and use of data across agencies and departments. These requirements are already showing tangible impacts for data users and researchers. For example, the HHS Statistical Official has led efforts to improve metadata and apply consistent tagging and digital object identifiers to their data sets, increasing the discoverability and usability of their data assets.

The Evidence Act also required OMB to establish "one front door" leading users to government data assets. In launching Researchdatagov.org, with its growing index of government data sets available for research, agencies have taken a big step forward in democratizing data access. Before this site launched, those seeking federal government data sets had to contact individual agencies and navigate their separate application processes. The catalog in

AJPH December 2023, Vol 113, No. 12

Researchdatagov.org further helps researchers and policymakers understand where current data gaps exist.

Agencies are also helping researchers discover data equity resources. For example, the HHS Assistant Secretary for Planning and Evaluation highlights demographic and economic characteristics to support analyses of health disparities, as seen in the inventory[17] of products resulting from the Patient-Centered Outcomes Research Trust Fund and the HHS-wide inventory[18] of federal data for conducting patient-centered outcomes research on economic outcomes.

Addressing the recommendation of the Equitable Data Working Group to provide tools that help users analyze and navigate data, the Census Bureau has released multiple data equity tools[19] that illustrate digital equity, economic mobility, community resilience, and more. The Census Bureau has also developed data products that inform studies about social determinants of health, including demographic portraits[20] of Supplemental Nutrition Assistance Program recipients, an interactive tool for analyzing small-area income and poverty estimates by age,[21] and My Community Explorer,[22] which provides economic, social, race and ethnicity, and business profiles through a user-friendly, interactive map. These resources, data inventories, and tools alike enable users to more easily find, explore, and compare data—making access to data more equitable.

The pandemic compelled federal agencies to reevaluate data infrastructures to address pressing policy challenges. New laws, including the Evidence Act described previously, and the Creating Helpful Incentives to Produce Semiconductors and Science Act of 2022[23] (CHIPS Act) facilitate the collection, maintenance, and evaluation of federal, state, local, territorial, and tribal data to strengthen capacity-building efforts. Specifically, the CHIPS Act establishes a National Secure Data Service (NSDS) demonstration project to show how a government-wide data linkage and privacy protection strategy could evolve and support researchers and equity assessments.

The Advisory Committee on Data for Evidence Building report,[24] released in October 2022, generated recommendations for how an NSDS could expand access to data, enable robust, accurate data linkages, and develop privacy-preserving techniques. The Committee recommended that the NSDS consider potential harms to vulnerable and marginalized populations when their data are used, specifically assessing the value of linkages and analyses relative to privacy concerns. An NCHS pilot (https://bit.ly/3Fltv9G) has been launched to determine promising uses for interoperable vital statistics, given the variation in unmet measurement needs across federal, state, and local levels. These needs are difficult to address because of chronic underinvestment in data infrastructure.

Federal agencies are investing in system modernizations to enable real-time data sharing with other federal agencies, state and local governments, and private and nonprofit data collectors. HHS has made strides toward interoperability at scale by establishing governance models within health information networks. HHS leadership on the Trusted Exchange Framework and Common Agreement (https://bit.ly/3tCgru5) focuses on transparency and privacy, which are critical for health data equity.

ADVANCING EQUITABLE METHODS

Federal agencies are actively exploring how artificial intelligence (AI) and machine learning can be used responsibly to ensure more ethical and equitable uses of federal health data. Current efforts include HHS's development of a Trustworthy AI (https://bit.ly/46t7Ubc) playbook to reduce risks and build public trust when applying AI in federal activities and the National Cancer Institute's encouragement of greater attention to data bias (https://bit.ly/46zTeHg) when employing AI. NCHS is also increasing its use of AI; they currently employ AI tools in survey operations for nonresponse detection, to code cause of death using text strings (https://www.cdc.gov/nchs/nvss/medcoder.htm), and to identify and replace personally identifiable information provided in interviews using speech-to-text software. These efforts result in greater efficiency and better data quality.

HHS also leads in research on using privacy-enhancing technologies that reduce risks of disclosure for groups and individuals in data sets. Privacy-preserving data linkages have been tested and implemented in the National COVID Cohort Collaborative (https://ncats.nih.gov/n3c), National Institutes of Health's All of Us[25] program, and NCHS's linkage (https://bit.ly/3QkEoig) of the National Hospital Care Survey with Medicaid data. Federal investment in high-risk, high-reward projects is developing through the Advanced Research Projects Agency for Health (ARPA-H; https://arpa-h.gov). Following other ARPAs, ARPA-H will invite both public and private organizations to design innovative solutions to complex problems. This represents a major shift in how federal agencies fund medical research, supporting the next generation of moonshots for health, advancing both science and the awareness of diversity and equity issues. We look forward to seeing how ARPA-H can accelerate secure, responsible health surveillance and AI-enabled solutions to reduce disease burdens and find cures.

It is also worth noting where federal policies spur changes among providers and health information systems. In 2024, CMS (https://bit.ly/48Yt4je) and many states will require hospitals to implement SDOH screenings for all patients aged 18 years and older, thereby creating a consistent collection of standardized data that various agencies can use. Many vendors offer the ability to collect data on these social factors (https://bit.ly/3Q20B38) that influence health status but are not directly medical, through standardized, structured data fields (i.e., Z-codes). SDOH indicators range from housing stability to social connectedness. Information can be collected during clinical encounters by providers, social workers, community health workers, case managers, patient navigators, and nurses through health risk assessments, screening tools, and self-reporting. The Joint Commission (https://bit.ly/3S28CIc) and the National Committee for Quality Assurance created requirements and reimbursement incentives to collect richer SDOH data. Federal agencies could incentivize SDOH data collection—especially across Medicare Advantage, Medicaid, and commercial payers. Some providers are concerned about asking patients about their unmet housing, food, and safety needs without having adequate resources to provide them. To mitigate some of these concerns, the Centers for Disease Control and Prevention has provided grants (https://www.cdc.gov/populationhealth/sdoh/index.htm) to state, local, territorial, and tribal jurisdictions to implement cross-sector interventions that impact many of these social needs.

SUMMARY

We have highlighted numerous, ongoing federal initiatives and activities, including large-scale investments, major changes in data collection and access, and subtle but meaningful changes in processes.

Were you aware of these activities? If not, consider tracking research coming out of the Federal Committee on Statistical Methodology (https://www.fcsm.gov) and the NSDS demonstration project (https://ncses.nsf.gov/about/national-secure-data-service-demo#card1896) to stay informed on data standards and methods that improve equitable data access and uses.

Researchers and public health professionals need to engage with federal agencies to achieve a public health data system with complete and accurate data to identify and address inequities. We need to acknowledge the need to collect and use demographic characteristics that reveal unique aspects of our population. It is critical that all groups are visible, as they grow or shrink in number, and as they disperse across regions or cluster together. Among federal statistical agencies, there is tension between visibility and privacy for these groups. We need a constructive, open dialogue on resolving this tension to find balance between data privacy and utility. AJPH

CORRESPONDENCE

Correspondence should be sent to Amy O'Hara, 600 New Jersey Ave NW, Massive Data Institute, Washington, DC 20001 (e-mail: amy.ohara@georgetown.edu). Reprints can be ordered at https://ajph.org by clicking the "Reprints" link.

PUBLICATION INFORMATION

Full Citation: O'Hara A, Rhodes R. The federal agencies' hidden efforts to produce equitable data. *Am J Public Health*. 2023;113(12):1278–1282.

Acceptance Date: September 17, 2023.

DOI: https://doi.org/10.2105/AJPH.2023.307465

CONTRIBUTORS

Amy O'Hara and Rosemary Rhodes contributed to the design and conduct of this research, and to the writing of the article.

ACKNOWLEDGMENTS

This work was supported by the Robert Wood Johnson Foundation (grant #79331).

CONFLICTS OF INTEREST

The authors have no conflicts of interest to report.

REFERENCES

1. Advancing racial equity and support for underserved communities through the federal government. *Fed Regist.* 2021;86(7009):7009–7013.
2. Further advancing racial equity and support for underserved communities through the federal government. *Fed Regist.* 2023;88(10825):10825–10833.
3. Equitable Data Working Group. A vision for equitable data: recommendations from the Equitable Data Working Group. 2022. Available at: https://www.whitehouse.gov/wp-content/uploads/2022/04/eo13985-vision-for-equitable-data.pdf. Accessed June 21, 2023.
4. Initial proposals for updating OMB's race and ethnicity statistical standards. *Fed Regist.* 2023;88(5375):5375–5384.
5. US Census Bureau. Middle East/North Africa (MENA) reporting category. Available at: https://www2.census.gov/about/partners/cac/nac/meetings/2022-05/discussant-mena-reporting-category.pdf. Accessed June 15, 2023.
6. State of the nation's health data infrastructure: experts weigh in two years into pandemic. *Amstat News*. March 1, 2022. Available at: https://magazine.amstat.org/blog/2022/03/01/nchs. Accessed June 15, 2023.
7. Limburg A, Kurczewski, K, Udalova, V. Enhancing race and ethnicity information in Medicaid data: the role of Census Bureau data. US Census Bureau. February 2, 2023. Available at: https://www.census.gov/library/working-papers/2023/demo/SEHSD-WP2023-05.html. Accessed June 15, 2023.
8. Pillai D, Ndugga N, Artiga S. Health care disparities among Asian, Native Hawaiian, and other Pacific Islander (NHOPI) People. *KFF*. May 24, 2023. Available at: https://www.kff.org/racial-equity-and-health-policy/issue-brief/health-care-disparities-among-asian-native-hawaiian-and-other-pacific-islander-nhopi-people. Accessed June 15, 2023.
9. Federal Committee on Statistical Methodology. Measuring Sexual Orientation and Gender Identity Research Group. Available at: https://www.fcsm.gov/groups/sogi. Accessed June 15, 2023.
10. Office of the Chief Statistician of the United States. Recommendations on the best practices for the collection of sexual orientation and gender identity data on federal statistical surveys. Available at: https://www.whitehouse.gov/wp-content/uploads/2023/01/SOGI-Best-Practices.pdf. Accessed June 20, 2023.
11. Centers for Disease Control and Prevention. CCQDER. Featured projects. 2022. Available at:

https://www.cdc.gov/nchs/CCQDER/collaborate/Projects.htm. Accessed June 15, 2023.

12. Bee A, Mitchell J, Mittag N, et al. National Experimental Wellbeing Statistics Version 1. February 14, 2023. Available at: https://www.census.gov/content/dam/Census/library/working-papers/2023/demo/sehsd-wp2023-02.pdf. Accessed June 20, 2023.
13. Brown JD, Heggeness M, Dorinski S, Warren L, Yi M. Understanding the quality of alternative citizenship data sources for the 2020 census. June 2019. Available at: https://www2.census.gov/ces/wp/2018/CES-WP-18-38R.pdf. Accessed June 20, 2023.
14. US Census Bureau. Item allocation rates. Available at: https://www.census.gov/acs/www/methodology/sample-size-and-data-quality/item-allocation-rates. Accessed June 15, 2023.
15. Equitable Data Working Group. A Vision for Equitable Data: Recommendations from the Equitable Data Working Group. 2022.
16. Foundations for Evidence-Based Policymaking Act of 2018, 115th Congress (2019).
17. Assistant Secretary for Planning and Evaluation. OS-PCORTF Product Library. Available at: https://aspe.hhs.gov/collaborations-committees-advisory-groups/os-pcortf/os-pcortf-product-library. Accessed June 15, 2023.
18. Assistant Secretary for Planning and Evaluation. Data inventory: federal data for conducting patient-centered outcome research. Available at: https://aspe.hhs.gov/sites/default/files/documents/e91d7240a9155e053e5e26686a25d38c/Data-Inventory.pdf. Accessed June 15, 2023.
19. US Census Bureau. Data equity tools. Available at: https://www.census.gov/about/what/data-equity/tools.html. Accessed June 21, 2023.
20. US Census Bureau. Supplemental Nutrition Assistance Program (SNAP) eligibility & access. Available at: https://www.census.gov/library/visualizations/interactive/snap-eligibility-access.html. Accessed June 21, 2023.
21. US Census Bureau. Small Area Income and Poverty Estimates (SAIPE). Available at: https://www.census.gov/data-tools/demo/saipe/#. Accessed June 21, 2023.
22. US Census Bureau. My Community Explorer 2.4. Available at: https://experience.arcgis.com/experience/13a111e06ad242fba0fb62f25199c7dd. Accessed June 21, 2023.
23. CHIPS Act of 2022, 117th Cong, Pub L No. 117-167, 136 Stat 1372 (2022).
24. Bureau of Economic Analysis. Advisory Committee on Data for Evidence Building: Year 2 Report. October 14, 2022. Available at: https://www.bea.gov/system/files/2022-10/acdeb-year-2-report.pdf. Accessed June 15, 2023.
25. Kho AN, Yu J, Bryan MS, et al. Privacy-preserving record linkage to identify fragmented electronic medical records in the All of Us Research Program. In: Cellier P, Driessens K, eds. *Machine Learning and Knowledge Discovery in Databases - International Workshops of ECML PKDD 2019, Proceedings* (Communications in Computer and Information Science; Vol. 1168 CCIS). Cham, Switzerland: Springer; 2020:79–87. https://doi.org/10.1007/978-3-030-43887-6_7

Medi-Cal's Population Health Management Program: Advancing Shared Medicaid and Public Health Data Processes and Infrastructure

Sristi Sharma, MD, MPH, Palav Babaria, MD, MHS, David Tian, MD, MPP, and Linette Scott, MD, MPH

ABOUT THE AUTHORS

All authors are with the California Department of Health Care Services, Sacramento, CA.

See also Toward More Equitable Public Health Data, pp. 1276–1308.

Driving health equity and eliminating health disparities has been a core tenet for California's public programs. With more than 15 million people in California covered by Medi-Cal, the state's Medicaid program, there are approximately one in three individuals and one in two children and youths who receive health care through Medi-Cal.[1] The California Department of Health Care Services (DHCS), which administers Medi-Cal, has historically worked closely with state and local public health departments, including the California Department of Public Health (CDPH), to support data sharing and data infrastructure.

In January 2022, the DHCS embarked on a multiyear transformational set of initiatives called California Advancing and Innovating Medi-Cal (CalAIM) to transform health care, including launching a statewide population health management (PHM) program to introduce new benefits and services to promote whole-person care.[2] We highlight the existing DHCS and CDPH partnerships for data processes and infrastructure, key lessons learned, and how the collaboration will further support the CalAIM PHM program.

DATA SHARING

Although the scope of work done by DHCS and CDPH is different, both state departments form critical components of California's complex health care system. DHCS is the backbone of California's health care safety net and helps millions of low-income and disabled Californians with access to affordable, integrated, high-quality health care, including medical, dental, mental health, and long-term care and substance use treatment services. CDPH's fundamental responsibilities are comprehensive in scope and include infectious disease control and prevention, food safety, environmental health, laboratory services, patient safety, emergency preparedness, chronic disease prevention and health promotion, family health, health equity, and vital records and statistics. Despite the two distinct focuses of these departments, there are significant interactions and areas of synergy between them. These commonalities have formed the basis for establishing data-sharing frameworks between DHCS and CDPH to ensure data completeness and to improve outcomes for Medi-Cal members. We highlight two specific examples: blood lead screening and COVID-19 vaccinations.

DHCS and CDPH work together to monitor blood lead screening of children and the treatment of children with positive results for blood lead. For example, Medi-Cal and CDPH both conduct blood lead monitoring and interventions for children. CDPH, in collaboration with the local public health departments, conducts environmental assessments as well as testing and care coordination for children with lead exposure identified in blood tests. Consequently, CDPH focuses on the health of communities by identifying and mitigating exposure to lead and making sure treatment occurs. The Medi-Cal program requires all children to have blood lead screening tests at ages one and two years in accordance with federal and California regulations.[3]

DHCS reports these screening rates as part of annual federal Centers for Medicare and Medicaid Services (CMS) reporting requirements (form CMS-416) for the early and periodic screening, diagnostic, and treatment benefit.[4,5] Historically, the blood lead screening rate on the CMS-416 for children younger than six years who are covered by Medi-Cal has been less than the national average for children in Medicaid programs.[6] DHCS reporting through the CMS-416 is based

AJPH December 2023, Vol 113, No. 12

strictly on claims and encounter data submitted to DHCS. Recognizing that there may be limitations in claims and encounter data, DHCS partnered with CDPH, which maintains a statewide registry of blood lead tests and results for all children, to do an in-depth analysis. The departments were able to use the Interagency Data Exchange Agreement as the data-sharing agreement to support this work.[7]

After the execution of the data-sharing agreement, the departments were able to share and link data to assess a more accurate screening rate. A point-in-time analysis using Medi-Cal claims or encounters reported that approximately 55% of Medi-Cal members who were younger than three years were screened for blood lead levels in 2016.[8] When combined with CDPH registry data, DHCS reported approximately a 10% higher screening rate for Medi-Cal members compared with using Medi-Cal claims data alone.[8] In addition to identifying more accurate screening rates for Medi-Cal members, using the combined data reduces unnecessary duplicate testing for Medi-Cal members. Based on the initial analysis, the departments have continued to share data for monitoring and outreach, including sharing data with Medi-Cal managed care plans to improve screening and treatment of children in Medi-Cal. Lessons learned from this example include the importance of combining data sources to have a more complete understanding; data-sharing agreements, such as the Interagency Data Exchange Agreement; and relationships between departments to serve common populations.

Based on the lessons learned from the blood lead screening example in addition to other data sharing between DHCS and CDPH, the departments had processes for data sharing in place that could be used in response to the COVID-19 public health emergency. Specifically, DHCS and CDPH were able to use the existing data processes to quickly share COVID-19 vaccination data in a similar manner. Information from the California Immunization Registry, which CDPH maintains, were matched for Medi-Cal members for COVID-19 vaccinations. Similar to blood lead screening data, DHCS data included data only from Medi-Cal claims for the administration of the vaccine. Given the extensive federal funding for the vaccine, this resulted in claims representing a very small number of vaccinations for the Medi-Cal population. California Immunization Registry records included vaccination information from almost all locations that were providing COVID-19 vaccinations. Supplementing DHCS data with California Immunization Registry data demonstrated that Medi-Cal vaccination rates were significantly lower, sometimes as much as 30%, than the general population's rates.[9]

The data informed DHCS, and efforts were immediately redirected to improve vaccination rates among Medi-Cal members. Additionally, other disparities were analyzed, including using the vaccine equity metric developed by CDPH. Based on the shared data analysis, DHCS partnered and shared member-level information for COVID-19 vaccination uptake with managed care plans and other partners to facilitate improved and equitable outreach and accountability for COVID-19 vaccination services.[9] The shared COVID-19 vaccination rate data also informed state policies, and more than $350 million was allocated to equitable COVID-19 vaccination efforts across the state from 2021 through 2022 through a managed care plan incentive payment program.[10,11]

The incentive program encouraged managed care plans to track vaccination rates among their members through outreach efforts to underserved communities, establishment of data systems, and collaboration with state and local partners to ensure equitable access to COVID-19 vaccines. With this funding, the managed care plans conducted baseline assessments and follow-ups and identified targets and gaps for vaccination programs. At the conclusion of the incentive program, many managed care plans reported higher rates of vaccinations, some up to 18%, for their members.[12] Lessons learned from this example include the importance of building on previous experience, having comprehensive data to inform policy, and continued monitoring to document the impact of the policies.

POPULATION HEALTH MANAGEMENT PROGRAM

In DHCS, CalAIM is a set of initiatives with goals to (1) identify and manage the health care needs of Medi-Cal members through whole-person care approaches and social drivers of health; (2) improve quality outcomes, reduce health disparities, and transform the delivery system through value-based initiatives, modernization, and payment reform; and (3) decrease, for the enrollees, the complexity of navigation through the Medi-Cal system.[2] One of the key initiatives in CalAIM is the PHM, which provides an approach that includes processes such as data-driven risk stratification, predictive analytics, identification of gaps in care, and standardized assessment to identify Medi-Cal members' health needs and promote wellness.

The data are also used to prevent illness by understanding the risk of poor physical, behavioral, and social outcomes and providing appropriate services and supports. Through the program, members have efficient access to not just physical health care but also behavioral and oral health, long-term services and supports, and developmental and intellectual disabilities services. Given that close to 90% of Medi-Cal members are served by managed care plans, the CalAIM PHM program focuses on managed care plans to provide whole-system and person-centered services across the continuum of care.[1]

Managed care plans have previously evaluated the population's health and social needs in a fragmented manner that has resulted in siloed and incomplete data practices. Since the successful implementation of CalAIM, the PHM program requires the integration of data from various health and social departments. Lessons learned from data-sharing practices between DHCS and CDPH will be used. First, the managed care plans are directed to conduct a systematic and equitable population needs assessments in collaboration with the local health departments, including CDPH. Data from these assessments will be provided to DHCS on a regular basis and will be used for conducting data-driven risk stratification and predictive analytics to standardize health program assessment and identify community needs and gaps in care management, care coordination, and care transitions.

In addition, DHCS has been working directly with public health partners to address key components necessary for PHM program implementation, including new requirements effective January 2024 for shared responsibilities between managed care plans and local public health programs in memoranda of understanding, data-sharing processes for critical public health preventive services, and guidance to synergize analogous efforts of local managed care plans and public health departments.

Under the PHM program, DHCS and CDPH are working together to build on the existing data infrastructure and create new data integration opportunities for Medi-Cal members with public programs to address social drivers of health. This includes the development of memoranda of understanding templates that managed care plans will be able to use with local health departments and local Special Supplemental Nutrition Program for Women, Infants, and Children (WIC) program departments to maximize the enrollment of eligible individuals into WIC programs as early as possible during pregnancy. In the context of CalAIM, DHCS has received approval from CMS to fund health-related social needs through the Medi-Cal program with the condition that individuals eligible for other social programs, such as WIC, be served by those programs.[13]

This dual approach to data sharing and collaboration under the CalAIM PHM program decreases the duplication of data collection and increases the efficiency of health and social services programs in the various state departments. Furthermore, managed care plans, health care organizations, and the state will use these data to address whole-person health and social needs and to respond appropriately and in a data-driven manner to population health needs, including outbreaks and threats.

By supplementing traditional claims and encounter data with public health data (e.g., immunization registries, vital records, blood lead screening, and other registries), DHCS can get a more comprehensive picture of population gaps in care that do not rely on health care utilization alone, which is known to favor those who receive services. The data generated, including those for social drivers of health, will thus be comprehensive, equitable, and targeted toward measuring performance and quality metrics while complying with federal and state requirements. DHCS will further use the data to inform policies on health and social programs, public and stakeholder education, and quality improvement programs, including those designed to promote health equity among its members and increase the state's focus on health equity data.

CONCLUSIONS

DHCS and CDPH have collaborated for years to share data to improve services and health outcomes under specific preventive and public health programs for Medi-Cal members. In the process, the two departments have established a data-sharing infrastructure that can be quickly repurposed, as demonstrated by its recent use for COVID-19 vaccination record sharing during the pandemic. DHCS's CalAIM PHM program will now use and build on the existing data infrastructure to evaluate and improve population health outcomes for Medi-Cal members and to address disparities and health equity. AJPH

CORRESPONDENCE

Correspondence should be sent to Linette T. Scott, MD, MPH, Deputy Director & Chief Data Officer, Department of Health Care Services, Enterprise Data and Information Management, MS 2100, P.O. Box 997413, Sacramento, CA 95899-7413 (e-mail: Linette.Scott@dhcs.ca.gov). Reprints can be ordered at http://www.ajph.org by clicking the "Reprints" link.

PUBLICATION INFORMATION

Full Citation: Sharma S, Babaria P, Tian D, Scott L. Medi-Cal's population health management program: advancing shared Medicaid and public health data processes and infrastructure. *Am J Public Health*. 2023;113(12):1283–1286.

Acceptance Date: September 17, 2023.

DOI: https://doi.org/10.2105/AJPH.2023.307466

CONTRIBUTORS

S. Sharma and L. Scott wrote the first draft of the editorial. All authors supervised the study; conceptualized, reviewed, and edited the editorial; and approved the final version of the editorial.

ACKNOWLEDGMENTS

This project was funded by the California Department of Health Care Services (DHCS).

The authors would like to thank Laura Davidson for her contributions to the editing process. The authors also wish to acknowledge the DHCS employees, whose hard work and dedication is transforming the Medi-Cal program to ensure that Californians get the care they need to live healthier lives. Finally, the authors wish to acknowledge the ongoing partnership between the California Department of Public Health and Medi-Cal to support the Medi-Cal members.

Note. The contents of this editorial do not necessarily represent the official views or policies of the state of California.

CONFLICTS OF INTEREST

The authors have no conflicts of interest to declare.

REFERENCES

1. California Department of Health Care Services. Medi-Cal monthly eligible fast facts. 2023. Available at: https://www.dhcs.ca.gov/dataandstats/statistics/Documents/FastFacts-March2022.pdf. Accessed September 28, 2023.
2. California Department of Health Care Services. Medi-Cal transformation. 2022. Available at: https://www.dhcs.ca.gov/CalAIM/Pages/calaim.aspx. Accessed September 28, 2023.
3. California Department of Public Health. Standard of care on screening for childhood lead poisoning. Available at: https://www.cdph.ca.gov/Programs/CCDPHP/DEODC/CLPPB/Pages/screen_regs_3.aspx. Accessed September 28, 2023.
4. Centers for Medicare & Medicaid Services. CMS-416. Annual early and periodic screening, diagnostic and treatment (EPSDT) participation report. March 10, 2023. Available at: https://www.cms.gov/regulations-and-guidance/legislation/paperworkreductionactof1995/pra-listing-items/cms-416. Accessed September 12, 2023.
5. Centers for Medicare & Medicaid Services. Subpart B. Early and periodic screening, diagnosis, and treatment (EPSDT) of individuals under age 21. 1984. Available at: https://www.ecfr.gov/current/title-42/chapter-IV/subchapter-C/part-441/subpart-B. Accessed September 28, 2023.
6. Medicaid.gov. Early and periodic screening, diagnostic, and treatment. 2023. Available at: https://www.medicaid.gov/medicaid/benefits/early-and-periodic-screening-diagnostic-and-treatment/index.html. Accessed September 28, 2023.
7. Interagency Data Exchange. Interagency Data Exchange (IDEA) guidebook. August 24, 2022. Available at: https://docs.data.ca.gov/interagency-data-exchange-idea-guidebook. Accessed September 28, 2023.
8. California Department of Public Health. Blood lead screening rates for a cohort of California children served by Medi-Cal: a joint report from the California Department of Public Health-Department of Health Care Services. 2017. Available at: https://www.cdph.ca.gov/Programs/CCDPHP/DEODC/CLPPB/CDPH%20Document%20Library/CDPH-DHCS_Cohort_Analysis.pdf. Accessed September 28, 2023.
9. California Department of Health Care Services. Medi-Cal COVID-19 vaccines. 2023. Available at: https://www.dhcs.ca.gov/Pages/COVID-19-Vaccines.aspx. Accessed September 28, 2023.
10. Office of Governor Gavin Newsom. Governor Newsom proposes 2021–22 state budget. January 8, 2021. Available at: https://www.gov.ca.gov/2021/01/08/governor-newsom-proposes-2021-22-state-budget. Accessed September 28, 2023.
11. California Department of Health Care Services. Medi-Cal COVID-19 vaccination incentive program. March 7, 2022. Available at: https://www.dhcs.ca.gov/Documents/COVID-19/APL-21-010-Vaccine-Incentive.pdf. Accessed September 28, 2023.
12. California Department of Health Care Services. Ending the pandemic through equitable vaccine administration. 2021. Available at: https://www.gov.ca.gov/wp-content/uploads/2021/03/Equitable-Vaccine-Administration-Fact-Sheet.pdf. Accessed September 28, 2023.
13. Centers for Medicare & Medicaid Services. California CalAIM demonstration. 2023. Available at: https://www.medicaid.gov/medicaid/section-1115-demo/demonstration-and-waiver-list/81046. Accessed September 28, 2023.

Advancing Sexual and Gender Minority Population Health Using Electronic Health Record Data

Kellan E. Baker, PhD, MPH, Eleanor Sarkodie, MPH, Jennafer Kwait, PhD, MHS, Caroline Medina, MPA, MHS, Asa Radix, PhD, MPH, and Risa Flynn

ABOUT THE AUTHORS

Kellan E. Baker, Eleanor Sarkodie, Jennafer Kwait, and Caroline Medina are with Whitman-Walker Institute, Washington, DC. Asa Radix is with Callen-Lorde Community Health Center, New York, NY. Risa Flynn is with the Los Angeles LGBT Center, Los Angeles, CA.

See also Toward More Equitable Public Health Data, pp. 1276–1308.

The importance of sexual orientation and gender identity (SOGI) data in identifying and reducing health disparities has received increasing national attention in the United States over the past 10 years, resulting in more widespread collection of these data in population surveys, public health surveillance, administrative data systems, and electronic health records (EHRs).[1–3] These data have helped identify disparities related to sexual orientation and gender identity pertaining to critical public health concerns, such as mental and behavioral health conditions, exposure to violence, COVID-19 incidence, HIV prevention and treatment needs, cancer-screening rates, and tobacco use.[1]

These health inequities require evidence-informed public health interventions at the local, state, and national levels to protect and promote the health of sexual and gender minority (SGM) populations nationwide. They also point to the need for comprehensive data sets that permit data disaggregation to further investigate SGM disparities in relation to age and specific SGM identities (e.g., people who identify as queer, asexual, or pansexual) and robust intersectional analyses of inequities affecting SGM people with multiple marginalized identities, such as SGM people with disabilities and SGM people of color.[4]

The SGM population in the United States is growing: as of 2022, a little more than 7% (roughly 14 million people) of US adults identified as LGBTQ (lesbian, gay, bisexual, transgender/-sexual, queer or questioning). Still, however, few public health surveys and other data collection instruments consistently include SOGI measures.[4,5] These data gaps demand innovative approaches to gathering, analyzing, and using SOGI data for public health purposes. At the same time, particularly in the ongoing aftermath of the COVID-19 pandemic, jurisdictions across the United States are increasingly aware of the need to enhance the quality, availability, and utility of a broad array of public health data. Many of these efforts, including electronic case reporting and the Data Modernization Initiative through the Centers for Disease Control and Prevention, focus on EHRs as a rich potential source of information about individual- and population-level demographics, exposures associated with health risks, treatment and care utilization patterns, and health outcomes. These initiatives have the ability both to make public health surveillance timelier and more comprehensive and to help bridge the lingering chasm between public health and clinical medicine.

Achieving the full promise of EHR data for both US public health purposes and SGM population health improvement requires addressing the many obstacles that remain in the collection and use of valid SOGI data in EHRs. A baseline challenge is that many health care institutions historically do not collect SOGI data or attempt to identify SGMs among their patient populations. This is changing as understandings of health disparities have evolved, and barriers to SOGI data collection have now increasingly shifted toward operational challenges related to the collection of these data in practice. Another key challenge is missing or inadequate data caused by factors such as data collectors' refusal to ask SOGI questions; respondents choosing not to respond, particularly when limited response options do not reflect their identities; and inaccurate or vague SOGI categories, such as "other," "something else," or "not sure."[2,5,6]

But even when SOGI data are available at individual institutions, inconsistent definitions of key terms across health care organizations and EHR systems limit the ability to consolidate and harmonize data from multiple institutions, reducing the sample size and power of data from aggregate SGM cohorts that can be used to support evidence-based interventions. To address this limitation, federal and public health agencies must take greater action to understand and enhance SOGI data interoperability. Interoperability—that is, ensuring that EHR systems can communicate with each other, exchange data, and use data that have been exchanged—is essential for the creation of data sets with sufficient SGM patient numbers to permit meaningful population and public health usage.[7]

CURRENT GUIDELINES FOR DATA INTEROPERABILITY

The US Department of Health and Human Services has developed and maintains two guidelines that facilitate EHR data interoperability across the US health care industry: the Interoperability Standards Advisory and the US Core Data for Interoperability (USCDI), both overseen by the Office of the National Coordinator for Health Information Technology. The Interoperability Standards Advisory, first issued in 2015, provides a list of standards and implementation specifications to facilitate interoperability among health entities for clinical, public health, and research purposes.[8] It is intended to help health information technology system designers and implementers identify broadly accepted data standards that promote the easy exchange of information between entities.

First implemented in 2020, the USCDI is a curated set of health data classes and elements that establishes a baseline for which data must be exchangeable between entities for a wide range of uses.[9] Version 1 of the USCDI had no SOGI data elements; however, SOGI data have been included beginning with version 2 in 2021.[9] In effect, the USCDI lays out the requirement that SOGI data collected in EHRs can be exchanged, whereas the Interoperability Standards Advisory provides an overview of the terminology that can be used to effectuate that requirement. The USCDI and Interoperability Standards Advisory, which are frequently updated, provide clear direction for the standardized electronic exchange of EHR data, including SOGI data, and lay a foundation for systemized capture and use of these data.[9]

The Bureau of Primary Health Care in the Health Resources and Services Administration also provides standardized guidance on SOGI data collection. The bureau funds more than 1500 federally qualified health centers and look-alike clinics in underserved communities around the country through its Health Center Program.[10] Health centers in the program are required to provide Health Resources and Services Administration with standardized information about important metrics, such as patient characteristics, services provided, and health outcomes, on a yearly basis via the Uniform Data System.[10] The Uniform Data System began including SOGI data elements as a reporting requirement in 2016, and the Health Resources and Services Administration provides definitions for each SOGI category to guide how data should be reported; the definitions were most recently updated in 2018.[11]

CHALLENGES AND OPPORTUNITIES

Although progress has been made in recent years to improve the collection, analysis, and reporting of SOGI data to shape clinical and public health interventions, we are now at an especially critical juncture for this work. In 2022, at the behest of the National Institutes of Health, the National Academies of Sciences, Engineering, and Medicine released a report outlining the methodological evidence for measuring sexual orientation, gender identity, and sex. The report provides recommendations for best practices and specific measures to be used in surveys and research, administrative, and clinical and other health settings.[5] The Indian Health Service recently announced that it will add SOGI fields to its EHR system, and states are increasingly enacting laws to incorporate SOGI measures into public health data systems.[12,13]

Additionally, the Biden–Harris Administration has provided policymakers across all levels of government with a suite of tools that can be used to improve SOGI data collection in health care settings and beyond. For instance, Executive Order 14075, issued in June 2022, requires federal agencies to promote inclusive and responsible SOGI data collection and resulted in the 2023 Federal Evidence Agenda on LGBTQI+ Equity.[14] The executive order also requires federal agencies to develop and implement SOGI data action plans detailing how they will use SOGI data to advance equity for LGBTQI+ (lesbian, gay, bisexual, transgender/-sexual, queer or questioning, intersex, and all subsects) populations as outlined by the Federal Evidence Agenda.[14]

As the federal government continues to expand SOGI data collection requirements that promote evidence-based policymaking and advance health equity for SGM communities, there are multiple opportunities for the Department of Health and Human Services in particular to take action to enhance SOGI data interoperability. For example, as the Office of the National Coordinator for Health Information Technology continues to update the USCDI, it can maintain the requirement that certified EHR systems use a specific standard (e.g., SNOMED CT) to capture SOGI data. To ensure that the required standard includes up-to-date terminology and does not retain outdated and potentially offensive terms such as "homosexual," "female-to-male," or "male-to-female," standard developers can look to examples such as the Gender Harmony Project's collaborative efforts to update health level 7 terminology to align with both clinically useful and culturally appropriate concepts of sex and gender.[15]

The National Institutes of Health has released notices of funding opportunities to explore methodological advances in the collection of SOGI data; more research efforts should look specifically at SOGI data capture and exchange in and across EHR systems. As part of the Centers for Disease Control and Prevention's Data Modernization Initiative, it is also critical that the Department of Health and Human Services and state public health departments work together to enhance SOGI data collection, which may require migrating legacy data systems to participate in new data-sharing systems or the creation of new data infrastructure.

Interoperable SOGI data are key to building a more equitable public health system that effectively addresses health disparities for SGM populations. Consolidating and harmonizing data from multiple health care institutions offer the ability to increase the sample size and power of SGM cohorts that can drive investigations of health risks, needs, and outcomes in these communities. Public health agencies must take further action to address barriers to the interoperability and use of SOGI data in EHRs to realize the full potential of these data for both US public health purposes and SGM population health improvement. AJPH

CORRESPENDENCE

Correspondence should be sent to Eleanor Sarkodie, 1201 Sycamore Dr SE, Floor 5, Washington, DC 20032 (e-mail: esarkodie@whitman-walker.org). Reprints can be ordered at http://www.ajph.org by clicking the "Reprints" link.

PUBLICATION INFORMATION

Full Citation: Baker KE, Sarkodie E, Kwait J, Medina C, Radix A, Flynn R. Advancing sexual and gender minority population health using electronic health record data. *Am J Public Health*. 2023;113(12):1287–1289.

Acceptance Date: September 17, 2023.

DOI: https://doi.org/10.2105/AJPH.2023.307467

CONTRIBUTORS

K. E. Baker and E. Sarkodie co-led the writing. E. Sarkodie supervised the study. J. Kwait assisted with the study. All authors assisted with the writing.

ACKNOWLEDGMENTS

Support for this research comes from Wellspring Philanthropic Foundation.

We thank the clinics participating in the We Count Collaborative.

CONFLICTS OF INTEREST

None of the authors has any conflicts of interest to report.

REFERENCES

1. Cahill S, Grasso C, Keuroghlian A, Sciortino C, Mayer K. Sexual and gender minority health in the COVID-19 pandemic: why data collection and combatting discrimination matter now more than ever. *Am J Public Health*. 2020;110(9):1360–1361. https://doi.org/10.2105/AJPH.2020.305829
2. Grasso C, McDowell MJ, Goldhammer H, Keuroghlian AS. Planning and implementing sexual orientation and gender identity data collection in electronic health records. *J Am Med Inform Assoc*. 2019;26(1):66–70. https://doi.org/10.1093/jamia/ocy137
3. Eliason MJ, Streed CG Jr. Choosing "something else" as a sexual identity: evaluating response options on the National Health Interview Survey. *LGBT Health*. 2017;4(5):376–379. https://doi.org/10.1089/lgbt.2016.0206
4. Patterson JG, Jabson JM, Bowen DJ. Measuring sexual and gender minority populations in health surveillance. *LGBT Health*. 2017;4(2):82–105. https://doi.org/10.1089/lgbt.2016.0026
5. Becker T, Chin M, Bates N, ed. *Measuring Sex, Gender Identity, and Sexual Orientation*. Washington, DC: National Academies Press; 2022. https://doi.org/10.17226/26424
6. Jones JM. LGBT identification in US ticks up to 7.1%. February 17, 2022. Available at: https://news.gallup.com/poll/389792/lgbt-identification-ticks-up.aspx. Accessed July 3, 2023.
7. Mason C. Understand the four levels of interoperability in healthcare. September 22, 2023. Available at: https://www.wolterskluwer.com/en/expert-insights/understand-the-three-levels-of-interoperability. Accessed October 3, 2023.
8. HealthIT.gov. About the ISA. Available at: https://www.healthit.gov/isa/about-isa. Accessed January 21, 2022.
9. Department of Health and Human Services. HHS updates interoperability standards to support the electronic exchange of sexual orientation, gender identity and social determinants of health. July 9, 2021. Available at: https://www.healthit.gov/news/2021/7/9/hhs-updates-interoperability-standards-support-electronic-exchange-sexual-orientation. Accessed October 3, 2023.
10. Health Resources and Services Administration, Health Center Program. *Uniform Data System: 2023 Manual. Health Center Data Reporting Requirements*. Available at: https://bphc.hrsa.gov/sites/default/files/bphc/data-reporting/2023-uds-manual.pdf. Accessed July 3, 2023.
11. US Centers for Medicare & Medicaid Services. Uniform Data System (UDS). Years data system included sexual and gender minority (SGM)-related data elements: 2016–present. Available at: https://www.cms.gov/files/document/sgm-clearinghouse-uds.pdf. Accessed January 21, 2022.
12. Indian Health Service. Data capture of sexual orientation and gender identity. Available at: https://www.ihs.gov/ihm/circulars/2023/data-capture-of-sexual-orientation-and-gender-identity-information. Accessed June 27, 2023.
13. Network for Public Health Law. Sexual orientation and gender identity: improving health equity through better data collection. Available at: https://www.networkforphl.org/news-insights/sexual-orientation-and-gender-identity-improving-health-equity-through-better-data-collection. Accessed June 27, 2023.
14. National Science and Technology Council. Federal evidence agenda on LGBTQI+ equity. January 2023. Available at: https://www.whitehouse.gov/wp-content/uploads/2023/01/Federal-Evidence-Agenda-on-LGBTQI-Equity.pdf. Accessed January 26, 2023.
15. Baker KE, Compton D, Fechter-Leggett ED, Grasso C, Kronk CA. Will clinical standards not be part of the choir? Harmonization between the HL7 gender harmony project model and the NASEM measuring sex, gender identity, and sexual orientation report in the United States. *J Am Med Inform Assoc*. 2022;30(1):83–93. https://doi.org/10.1093/jamia/ocac205

Data Related to Social Determinants of Health Captured in the National Health and Nutrition Examination Survey

Denys T. Lau, PhD, Namanjeet Ahluwalia, PhD, DSc, Cheryl D. Fryar, MSPH, Matthew Kaufman, Irma E. Arispe, PhD, and Ryne Paulose-Ram, PhD, MA

ABOUT THE AUTHORS

All authors were with the National Center for Health Statistics, Centers for Disease Control and Prevention, Hyattsville, MD, when this work was conducted.

See also Toward More Equitable Public Health Data, pp. 1276–1308.

AJPH December 2023, Vol 113, No. 12

Health equity is defined as "attainment of the highest level of health for all people" and encompasses fair and just opportunities for everyone to be as healthy as possible.[1] Health equity research examines the existence of health disparities and their underlying factors, which can be categorized into broad determinants of health, including genetics, behavior, environmental influences, medical care, and social factors.[2] The last category, also known as social determinants of health (SDOH), includes social and structural factors, such as racism and discriminatory practices and policies.[3] *Healthy People 2030* categorizes SDOH into five domains[4]: education access and quality, economic stability, health care access and quality, social and community context, and neighborhood and built environment. Evidence shows that SDOH influence a wide range of health outcomes[5,6] and nutritional status.[7] Exposures to adverse SDOH, such as food deserts and unsafe neighborhoods, are inequitably experienced by subgroups that vary by race and ethnicity, socioeconomic status, and other characteristics historically associated with discrimination or exclusion. Variation among groups in access to resources and their differential vulnerability to adverse exposures result in health disparities.[8]

Collecting high-quality data on SDOH is an important part of the US Department of Health and Human Services' strategy for achieving health equity.[9] To identify health disparities, the National Center for Health Statistics (NCHS) prioritizes advancing health equity research through data collection and analysis related to social factors associated with health inequities. Conducted by NCHS, the National Health and Nutrition Examination Survey (NHANES) is a series of cross-sectional surveys that collect nationally representative data for adults and children in the United States.[10]

NHANES data are used to produce national estimates on disease prevalence, nutritional status, and environmental exposures. Distinct from other national surveys, NHANES collects multimode data through interviews, health examinations, and laboratory testing using a complex sampling design.[11] Since 1999, NHANES has operated continuously and released public use files for each two-year cycle with data for approximately 10 000 participants. An exception is the 2017 to March 2020 prepandemic data release, which combined the 2017 to 2018 cycle with the subsequent cycle that was suspended in March 2020 because of the COVID-19 pandemic. A full description of NHANES is available at www.cdc.gov/nchs/nhanes.

Given the importance of understanding the role of SDOH in health outcomes, we discuss the content and utility of NHANES as an important source of nationally representative data for supporting health equity research, especially studies examining SDOH. Specifically, we describe NHANES data collected on determinants of health related to genetics, behavior, and environmental influences, while emphasizing data captured on SDOH-related factors. Additionally, we describe NHANES' sociodemographic characteristic data, which can be used to characterize population subgroups with inequitable exposure to SDOH as well as NHANES' links to external data sources to expand contextual SDOH-related data. Finally, we discuss future opportunities that could enhance NHANES' capacity to contribute to SDOH research.

GENETICS, BEHAVIOR, AND ENVIRONMENT

NHANES has provided essential data for tracking our nation's progress toward meeting *Healthy People* and other public health objectives and measuring disparities in exposures, health conditions, and outcomes. NHANES data from dietary and health interviews, health examinations, and biospecimen testing (e.g., measurement of metabolites, inflammatory markers, antibody levels) are used to identify chronic conditions, infectious diseases, food intake and nutritional status, and toxic substance exposures.

Regarding genetics data, DNA was purified from blood collected in NHANES 1999 to 2002 and 2007 to 2012 and stored for future studies. The breadth of data collected in NHANES affords opportunities to assess associations among genetics, health conditions, disease, and SDOH.[12] Concerning behavioral determinants of health, since 1999, NHANES has collected self-reported data on diet behavior, physical activities, lifetime and current sexual behaviors, vaccination schedules, smoking and tobacco use, and alcohol and other drug use.[10]

Regarding environmental determinants of health, earlier cycles of NHANES collected household samples of dust and water as objective measures of housing characteristics. From 1999 to 2006, dust samples were obtained to determine the presence of lead and indoor allergens.[13] From 1999 to 2010, household tap water samples were tested for volatile organic compounds and, in 2013 to 2016, for fluoride. Besides household sample collection, NHANES continuously collects blood and urine samples of respondents to test for a multitude of chemicals to determine environmental exposures at the individual level. In addition, respondents reported subjective measures of housing conditions and work environments during household interviews. Additional data on environmental exposures can be linked to NHANES from external data sources.

RELATED FACTORS

Although SDOH encompass social, economic, and political factors that influence people's access to resources, individual characteristics are important for stratifying populations to examine the exposure to and impact of SDOH. NHANES collects data about individual characteristics that are related to SDOH. The NHANES household interview collects self-reported data on personal characteristics that are related to the *Healthy People 2030* SDOH framework[4]: education access and quality, economic stability, health care access and quality, social and community context, and neighborhood and built environment. Appendixes A to C (available as a supplement to the online version of this article at http://www.ajph.org) summarize key SDOH-related data that have been collected and publicly released for each NHANES cycle from 1999 to 2000.

To determine educational attainment of adults and children aged 6 years and older, NHANES asks participants the highest education level they have completed (Appendix A). Regarding economic stability, NHANES asks respondents about their annual and monthly family income. NHANES provides the ratio of family income to poverty level by dividing family income by the federal poverty threshold.[14] Since 1999, respondents reported income received from government financial subsidies such as Social Security or disability pensions. Respondents are asked about their homeownership, occupation, work schedules, and reasons for unemployment.

Since 1999, NHANES has collected information on food security status using the US Food Security Survey Module; however, questions at the individual level were added from 2003 to 2010 asking about personal experience with not having enough money to buy food. Since 1999, respondents in all cycles reported whether they recently received or were currently receiving benefits from the Supplemental Nutrition Assistance Program; the Special Supplemental Nutrition Program for Women, Infants, and Children; or school meal assistance. Since 2003, respondents reported meals received from home-delivery programs or other emergency meal sources.

The NHANES interview gathers detailed data on health care access (Appendix B). From 1999 to 2004, respondents reported whether their health insurance covered dental care and, since 2005, whether prescription drugs were covered. Respondents reported their usual source of health care. Unmet need for dental care was collected in the 2003 to 2004 and again in the 2011 to 2012 cycles.

Regarding social and community context, from 1999 to 2008, NHANES asked adult respondents whether they could count on someone for emotional or financial support (Appendix C), who provided this support, and whether they could have used more support. Additionally, respondents provided information on their neighborhood and built environment. From 1999 to 2018, respondents reported the number of rooms in their home and the number of people residing in the household, which could be used to evaluate crowding. Earlier cycles of NHANES asked respondents about the condition of paint (1999–2004) and the presence of mildew and cockroaches and other pests inside the home (2005–2006). Since 2007, exposure to volatile organic compounds from household products was reported. All survey cycles collected information on respondents' recent exposures to secondhand smoke at home and the workplace, with questions about exposures to tobacco smoke in cars and restaurants since 2013 and e-cigarettes since 2017. All cycles, except 2013 to 2014, contained questions on noise exposure and use of protective hearing devices at work. From 2007 to 2012, respondents were asked about their exposures at work to dusts, exhaust, and other fumes.

SOCIODEMOGRAPHIC CHARACTERISTICS

NHANES collects data on respondents' sociodemographic characteristics that can be used to stratify populations to examine inequitable exposure to SDOH (Box 1).[8] Since 1999, NHANES has collected data on race and Hispanic origin using the following categories: Mexican American, non-Hispanic Black, non-Hispanic White, Hispanic other, and other racial groups. An "all Hispanic" category including Mexican American and other Hispanic groups was added in 2007, and a non-Hispanic Asian category was added in 2011.

Questions on sexual orientation have been included since 2001. Respondents' country of birth (nativity) was collected and publicly released as "born in the 50 states" (i.e., 50 states and Washington, DC) or "outside of the 50 states," originally separating only Mexico as an option, then expanding in 2007 to all Spanish-speaking countries, and finally simplifying in 2011 to "outside the 50 states." Other acculturation data included citizenship (until 2018), language spoken, and number of years living in the United States. Until 2018, respondents' physical functioning in activities of daily living were collected. Questions on disability status, such as difficulty in seeing, hearing, and walking, were added in 2013.

NHANES oversampled certain subpopulations to increase the reliability of estimates for subgroups. The increased reliability of estimates supports the examination of inequitable distribution of SDOH among subpopulations.[11,15] Appendix D (available as a supplement to the online version of this article at http://www.ajph.org) summarizes oversampling in NHANES from 1999 to March 2020. In 1999 to 2006, Mexican American and non-Hispanic Black populations were oversampled. Oversampling changed from 2007 to 2010, with the entire Hispanic population being oversampled rather than only the Mexican American subgroup. This oversampling approach made it possible to

BOX 1— Sociodemographic Characteristics Interview Items in the National Health and Nutrition Examination Survey Public Use Data Files by Survey Period: United States, 1999–March 2020

Race and Hispanic origin	1999–2006: Mexican American, non-Hispanic White, non-Hispanic Black, other Hispanic, other race (including multiracial). 2007–2010: All Hispanic category added (Mexican American, other Hispanic); beginning of oversampling of all Hispanic people. 2011–March 2020: Non-Hispanic Asian category added; beginning of oversampling of non-Hispanic Asian people.
Sexual orientation	2001–2016: Sexual orientation.
Marital/relationship status	1999–March 2020: Categories: married, widowed, divorced, separated, never married, living with partner.
Nativity	1999–2006: Born in the US, Mexico, or another country. 2007–2010: Born in the US, Mexico, a Spanish-speaking country (not Mexico), or a non–Spanish-speaking country outside the US. 2011–March 2020: Born in or outside the US.
Citizenship[a]	1999–2018: US citizenship status.
Language	1999–2004: Language read and spoken, used as child, used to think, and used with friends. 2003–March 2020: Languages respondent used and interpreter used during interviews. 2005–March 2020: Usual language spoken at home.
Years living in the US	1999-March 2020: Length of time in the US.
Disability status/physical functioning[a]	1999–2018: Physical functioning questions on limitations in instrumental activities of daily living (e.g., balancing a checkbook, grocery shopping) and activities of daily living (e.g., getting in and out of bed). 2013–2018: Disability questions on difficulty with seeing, hearing, walking, dressing, concentrating, and running errands.

Note. Periods are 1999–2000, 2001–2002, 2003–2004, 2005–2006, 2007–2010, 2011–2012, 2013–2016, and 2017–March 2020. The National Health and Nutrition Examination Survey (NHANES) data collected 1999–2018 have been released in two-year cycles. Cycles with the same survey content are combined in the same columns. In addition to data released for the 2017–2018 cycle, a separate nationally representative sample of NHANES 2017–March 2020 prepandemic data were released, which combined data collected from the 2017–2018 and 2019–March 2020 cycles. Beginning in 2017, data on sexual orientation have been available only in the National Center for Health Statistics Research Data Center.

[a]Data on citizenship and on disability status/physical functioning were released in public use data files through the 2017–2018 cycle, but these data from the 2017–March 2020 prepandemic files are available only through the Research Data Center.

produce reliable estimates for the entire Hispanic population since 2007. From 2011 to March 2020, NHANES also oversampled the non-Hispanic Asian population. Oversampling also has been based on age and income status.[10]

To improve language access for some racial and ethnic minorities, NHANES is conducted in English or Spanish based on respondent preference, with translators available for other languages. In 2011 to 2018, to facilitate oversampling of Asian individuals, selected survey materials were translated into Mandarin Chinese, Korean, and Vietnamese.[16]

DATA LINKAGE WITH NHANES

Data sources linked to NHANES through the NCHS Data Linkage Program expanded the availability of variables for SDOH research by providing additional information on SDOH and other exposures and outcomes. Only survey participants who have provided consent and have the necessary personally identifiable information are included in person-level links. NHANES data have been linked to data from the Centers for Medicare & Medicaid Services; the US Renal Data System; the Department of Housing and Urban Development; and the Department of Veterans Affairs.[17] A sample of publications using linked data is available on the NCHS Web site. Additionally, NHANES data have been linked to mortality data from the National Death Index. Information from NHANES and death certificates of survey participants can support research on the association between SDOH and mortality.[18,19]

Linking data sources increases the information available for analysis and adds a longitudinal component to the surveys by providing multiple years of administrative data. For example, linked NHANES and Centers for Medicare & Medicaid Services data add information on health care use and cost over time.[20] To protect respondents' confidentiality, most NHANES linked data files must be accessed through the Research Data Center. However, public use files are available for 1999 to 2018 NHANES data linked with mortality data through 2019 (https://bit.ly/46WrooF).

Although the Data Linkage Program develops files that directly link survey respondents with administrative data, researchers can also examine SDOH by merging external sources of contextual data with NHANES data using geographic information.[21] Merged data can offer insights into respondents' community context, such as availability of grocery stores and health care providers, public safety of the built environment, and environmental characteristics. Examples of contextual-level data sources are available in the Agency for Healthcare Research and Quality SDOH Database (https://bit.ly/46zgLrQ). Merging contextual data with NHANES data files must be done through the Research Data Center.

FUTURE OPPORTUNITIES

Future opportunities to increase NHANES' capacity to advance SDOH research include adding new or removed SDOH-related items and biomarkers, including indoor samples related to housing quality, and expanding data links. For each survey cycle, NHANES considers input from external stakeholders on new or expanded content based on respondent burden, available funding, and public health significance.[10] As the current NHANES cycle completes its fielding in fall 2023, the next iteration of the survey is being redesigned.

New or removed SDOH-related items are being considered for inclusion on the household interview survey. For example, NCHS recently added perceived discrimination, social support, and loneliness measures to the National Health Interview Survey. NHANES could add these questions to assess their relationships with measured biological factors and other health indicators. NCHS is also evaluating approaches to better assess gender identity in future NHANES cycles and other surveys. Additionally, increasing the number of biomarkers of stress, such as allostatic load measures, is being evaluated. However, adding SDOH-related questions to NHANES creates challenges, such as balancing respondent burden and decreasing response rates. Many SDOH-related measures have not been psychometrically validated or tested in national surveys.

Indoor sample collection could be evaluated for future cycles to objectively measure home environmental exposures, water quality, and housing quality. Challenges to indoor sample collection include increased survey costs and resources as well as participants' privacy concerns. Besides household sample collection, blood and urine samples of respondents that NHANES continuously collects are analyzed for various environmental chemical exposures at the individual level.

Because NHANES has a relatively small sample size owing to operational costs, generating reliable estimates for small subgroups remains a challenge. NHANES has oversampled subgroups by race, Hispanic origin, age, and income to increase their sample sizes and thereby improve the statistical reliability of estimates for subgroups. However, oversampling subgroups may not guarantee sufficient sample sizes. One implementation challenge of oversampling is increased survey costs. Additionally, concerted efforts to build trust, address barriers to participation, and value community expertise are warranted to help ensure meaningful engagement with subgroups, especially those who have historically been disadvantaged.[22]

Causal research studies are challenging because of NHANES's cross-sectional design. To enhance trend assessment and causal inference of SDOH's impact on health disparities, NHANES could consider longitudinal follow-up with survey participants. However, implementing a longitudinal survey design leads to resource constraints and attrition rates in sequential survey waves.

The NCHS Data Linkage Program is working to expand the number and types of external data sources linked to NHANES and to increase researcher access to linked data files while still protecting participant confidentiality. For example, the Data Linkage Program is evaluating the use of privacy-preserving record linkage as a strategy to expand the data sources that could be linked to NHANES. NCHS is launching its virtual data enclave to increase researcher access outside the Research Data Center by allowing remote access to restricted use data, including linked data files.

CONCLUSIONS

Nationally representative data collected during NHANES interviews, health examinations, and biospecimen collection support health equity research, including studies examining SDOH. NHANES collects data on determinants of health related to genetics, behavior, and environmental influences, as well as SDOH-related data, including education, economic stability, health care, social and community context, and neighborhood or built environment. Survey design elements such as oversampling may allow the expanded analyses of subgroups disproportionately exposed to adverse SDOH. Linking to external data sources increases contextual information to enable additional analyses. Future opportunities to increase NHANES' capacity to contribute to SDOH research include additional SDOH-related items, indoor sampling, and data linkage expansion. For the opportunities identified, implementation challenges will need to be evaluated, such as increased costs, limited validated measures, and increased respondent burden. AJPH

CORRESPONDENCE

Correspondence should be sent to Denys T. Lau, PhD, 3311 Toledo Rd, Hyattsville, MD 20782 (e-mail: wyr1@cdc.gov). Reprints can be ordered at http://www.ajph.org by clicking the "Reprints" link.

PUBLICATION INFORMATION

Full Citation: Lau DT, Ahluwalia N, Fryar CD, Kaufman M, Arispe IE, Paulose-Ram R. Data related to social determinants of health captured in the National Health and Nutrition Examination Survey. *Am J Public Health*. 2023;113(12):1290–1295.

Acceptance Date: September 30, 2023.

DOI: https://doi.org/10.2105/AJPH.2023.307490

CONTRIBUTORS

D. T. Lau supervised the work. D. T. Lau, N. Ahluwalia, C. D. Fryar, M. Kaufman, and I. E. Arispe drafted the article. D. T. Lau, N. Ahluwalia, C. D. Fryar, and I. E. Arispe conceptualized the work. All authors revised and approved the article.

ACKNOWLEDGMENTS

The authors sincerely thank the following for their help in reviewing earlier versions of this article and validating its content: Steven Fink, Jody McLean, Lisa Mirel, and the project officers of the Division of Health and Nutrition Examination Surveys at the National Center for Health Statistics.

Note. The findings and conclusions in this work are those of the authors and do not necessarily represent the views of the Centers for Disease Control and Prevention.

CONFLICTS OF INTEREST

We have no potential or actual conflicts of interests from funding or affiliation-related activities to report.

REFERENCES

1. US Department of Health and Human Services. Health equity and health disparities environmental scan. March 2022. Available at: https://health.gov/sites/default/files/2022-04/HP2030-HealthEquityEnvironmentalScan.pdf. Accessed June 30, 2023.
2. Centers for Disease Control and Prevention. Social determinants of health. Frequently asked questions. 2019. Available at: https://www.cdc.gov/nchhstp/socialdeterminants/faq.html. Accessed June 30, 2023.
3. Hacker K, Houry D. Social needs and social determinants: the role of the Centers for Disease Control and Prevention and public health. *Public Health Rep*. 2022;137(6):1049–1052. https://doi.org/10.1177/00333549221120244
4. US Department of Health and Human Services. *Healthy People 2030*. Social determinants of health. Available at: https://health.gov/healthypeople/priority-areas/social-determinants-health#:~:text=How%20Does%20Healthy%20People%202030,well%2Dbeing%20for%20all.%E2%80%9D. Accessed June 30, 2023.
5. McGovern L, Miller G, Hughes-Cromwick P. Health policy brief: the relative contribution of multiple determinants to health outcomes. *Health Affairs*. August 21, 2014. Available at: https://www.healthaffairs.org/do/10.1377/hpb20140821.404487/full/healthpolicybrief_123-1687440743592.pdf. Accessed September 25, 2023.
6. Park Y, Mulligan N, Gleize M, et al. Discovering associations between social determinants and health outcomes: merging knowledge graphs from literature and electronic health data. *AMIA Annu Symp Proc*. 2022;2021:940–949. Available at: https://www.ncbi.nlm.nih.gov/pmc/articles/PMC8861749. Accessed October 24, 2023.
7. US Department of Agriculture and US Department of Health and Human Services. *Dietary Guidelines for Americans, 2020–2025*. 9th ed. December 2020. Available at: https://www.dietaryguidelines.gov/sites/default/files/2020-12/Dietary_Guidelines_for_Americans_2020-2025.pdf. Accessed June 30, 2023.
8. Dahlgren G, Whitehead M. The Dahlgren–Whitehead model of health determinants: 30 years on and still chasing rainbows. *Public Health*. 2021;199:20–24. https://doi.org/10.1016/j.puhe.2021.08.009
9. De Lew N, Sommers BD. Addressing social determinants of health in federal programs. *JAMA Health Forum*. 2022;3(3):e221064. https://doi.org/10.1001/jamahealthforum.2022.1064
10. Centers for Disease Control and Prevention. National Health and Nutrition Examination Survey. Available at: https://www.cdc.gov/nchs/nhanes/index.htm. Accessed June 30, 2023.
11. Akinbam LJ, Chen TC, Davy O, et al. National Health and Nutrition Examination Survey, 2017–March 2020 prepandemic file: sample design, estimation, and analytic guidelines. *Vital Health Stat 1*. 2022;(190):1–36. https://doi.org/10.15620/cdc:115434
12. National Center for Health Statistics. National Health and Nutrition Examination Survey. DNA

Specimens and Genetic Data Program. Available at: https://www.cdc.gov/nchs/nhanes/biospecimens/dnaspecimens.htm. Accessed June 30, 2023.

13. Centers for Disease Control and Prevention. *National Health and Nutrition Examination Survey: Allergen Dust Collection Procedures Manual*. August 2006. Available at: https://www.cdc.gov/nchs/data/nhanes/nhanes_05_06/allergen_manual_06.pdf. Accessed June 30, 2023.
14. US Department of Health and Human Services. Prior Department of Health and Human Services' poverty guidelines and Federal Register references. Available at: https://aspe.hhs.gov/topics/poverty-economic-mobility/poverty-guidelines/prior-hhs-poverty-guidelines-federal-register-references. Accessed June 30, 2023.
15. Curtin LR, Mohadjer LK, Dohrmann SM, et al. National Health and Nutrition Examination Survey: sample design, 2007–2010. *Vital Health Stat* 2. 2013;(160):1–23. Available at: https://pubmed.ncbi.nlm.nih.gov/25090039. Accessed October 24, 2023.
16. Paulose-Ram R, Burt V, Broitman L, et al. Overview of Asian American data collection, release, and analysis: National Health and Nutrition Examination Survey 2011–2018. *Am J Public Health*. 2017;107(6):916–921. https://doi.org/10.2105/AJPH.2017.303815
17. National Center for Health Statistics. NCHS linked data table. February 14, 2022. Available at: https://www.cdc.gov/nchs/data/datalinkage/LinkageTable.pdf. Accessed June 30, 2023.
18. Banerjee S, Radak T, Khubchandani J, et al. Food insecurity and mortality in American adults: results from the NHANES-linked mortality study. *Health Promot Pract*. 2021;22(2):204–214. https://doi.org/10.1177/1524839920945927
19. Bush H, Paik J, Golabi P, et al. Impact of hepatitis C virus and insurance coverage on mortality. *Am J Manag Care*. 2019;25(2):61–67. Available at: https://pubmed.ncbi.nlm.nih.gov/30763036. Accessed October 24, 2023.
20. Mirel LB, Wheatcroft G, Parker JD, et al. Health characteristics of Medicare traditional fee-for-service and Medicare Advantage enrollees: 1999–2004 National Health and Nutrition Examination Survey linked to 2007 Medicare data. *Natl Health Stat Report*. 2012;(53):1–12. Available at: https://pubmed.ncbi.nlm.nih.gov/22808695. Accessed October 24, 2023.
21. Centers for Disease Control and Prevention. National Health and Nutrition Examination Survey (NHANES) geocodes. Available at: https://www.cdc.gov/rdc/geocodes/geowt_nhanes.htm#:~:text=National%20Health%20and%20Nutrition%20Examination%20Survey%20%28NHANES%29%20Geocodes,only%20available%20for%20adding%20contextual%20variables%20to%20NHANES. Accessed June 30, 2023.
22. Centers for Disease Control and Prevention. Meaningful community engagement for health and equity. Available at: https://www.cdc.gov/nccdphp/dnpao/health-equity/health-equity-guide/pdf/health-equity-guide/Health-Equity-Guide-sect-1-2.pdf. Accessed September 25, 2023.

Championing the 2021 New York State Law: A Step Toward Data Disaggregation on Asian Americans, Native Hawaiians, and Pacific Islanders

Anita Gundanna, PhD, Claudia M. Calhoon, DPH, Meeta Anand, JD, MA, Lloyd Feng, and Vanessa Leung, MA

ABOUT THE AUTHORS

Anita Gundanna, Lloyd Feng, and Vanessa Leung are with the Coalition for Asian American Children and Families, New York, NY. Claudia M. Calhoon is with the Department of Health and Human Performance, York College, City University of New York, New York. Meeta Anand is with The Leadership Conference on Civil and Human Rights, Washington, DC.

See also Toward More Equitable Public Health Data, pp. 1276–1308.

AJPH December 2023, Vol 113, No. 12

Racial and ethnic data aggregating Asian American and Native Hawaiian and Pacific Islander (AA and NH/PI) individuals into one or two categories do not provide an accurate picture of social needs or health outcomes among communities that identify as such.[1–4] Addressing these gaps in data is part of advancing data equity, which Lee et al. define as "a transparent, critically grounded approach to race and ethnicity data (dis)aggregation . . . necessary to document, understand, and address the health effects of racism."[5(p262)] Despite the long-standing acknowledgment of the gaps in AA and NH/PI population data, the passage of laws and changes in government data practices to correct these gaps have been slow.[4,6] New York City and State have taken important steps in collecting better data on the full range of AA and NH/PI populations. But the work to generate fully descriptive data that provide complete insights into health outcomes and social determinants and to support data equity remains incomplete.

In this article, we highlight the challenges of achieving data equity by advocating policies to fully disaggregate data, especially those that render invisible populations with heritage in Asia, Hawaii, and the Pacific Islands, through a detailed discussion of the Coalition for Asian American Children and Families (CACF) Invisible No More (INM) campaign in New York. Led by CACF, the decade-long INM campaign for AA and NH/PI data disaggregation led to the first-ever data disaggregation law in New York City in 2016, followed by the enactment of a New York State law in 2021. INM provides an important template for how coalition-based advocacy can successfully push for the passage and implementation of laws that mandate better data collection and usage.

In the United States, 21 million people identifying as AA and NH/PI make up 6% of the population.[7] Gaps in resources persist even though AA and NH/PI populations were the fastest-growing racial and ethnic minority group in the United States from 2000 to 2019.[8] In New York State, AA and NH/PI populations together make up more than 17% of the overall population.[9] Aggregated data on social determinants of health overstate the level of education, employment, and income among many populations that fall under this umbrella.[10] Such data also mask health disparities requiring public health intervention and social services.[10]

For example, aggregated data on COVID-19's impact on communities indicated that Asian Americans were the racial group least affected by COVID-19.[11–13] But research by New York University's Center for the Study of Asian American Health showed that at the height of the pandemic in 2020, Chinese New Yorkers suffered from the highest COVID-19 mortality rate and that South Asian New Yorkers had the highest infection and hospitalization rates across all New Yorkers.[11] Subsequently, aggregated community estimates pointed to high rates of vaccine uptake among AA and NH/PI communities overall.[14] Disaggregated data showed, however, that whereas vaccine acceptance among Nepali and Bangladeshi populations was high, vaccine uptake among these groups was relatively low, pointing to a missed opportunity for disease prevention.[14]

Effective data disaggregation for any population requires better infrastructure, practices, and procedures. In January 2023, the Office of Management and Budget issued initial proposed revisions to their policy directive that mandates how race and ethnicity data are collected at the federal level.[15] Notably, they included mandating data disaggregation that is more detailed than the five minimum race categories and the addition of a Middle Eastern North African category. New standards are expected to be announced by summer 2024.

Increased data disaggregation at the national level will help reinforce local and state efforts, especially toward harmonizing multiple systems and data sets. In the meantime, state and local efforts are where this battle is advanced in concrete ways. CACF's INM campaign provides a rich case study of a local effort seeking improved data disaggregation.

LESSONS AND RECOMMENDATIONS

For those seeking to advance this work in their state, we make the following recommendations.

Committing to This Work for the Long Term

Identifying allies, conducting public education, creating a demand for change, developing policy, and implementing changes take years. Community-based leadership with long institutional and programmatic memory requires sustained commitment and support from organization leadership and funders.

In 2009, New York State assembly member Grace Meng (D) first proposed an AA and NH/PI–focused state disaggregation law: it was signed into law in 2021. Concerted efforts to win a New York City law began in 2012 and went on until its passage in 2016. Work continues to monitor and advocate implementation that reflects data equity, as does work to revise legislation to address gaps in the initial laws. Governments, funders, and advocates must commit to a long fight for effective disaggregated data.

Moving Beyond a Scarcity Mindset

CACF found it important to address concerns that data disaggregation might lead to a diffusion of political power by creating divisions among different AA and NH/PI populations or by encouraging decision makers to focus on specific ethnic needs over shared needs.[16] CACF believes these fears are rooted in the harmful "model minority" myth, which casts Asian Americans as a monolithic group that neither needs social services nor experiences struggles.[15] To challenge these myths, CACF grounds their work in collective advocacy as well as the agency that AA and NH/PI communities have in continuing to advocate together. AA and NH/PI communities have depended on coalition-based advocacy across racial, ethnic, linguistic, and cultural differences to protect themselves from discrimination and to advocate government recognition of their needs.[17]

CACF focused on disaggregated data's revelation of inequities as—instead of a cause for division—an opportunity for AA and NH/PI communities to strengthen their collective advocacy; this was done by better understanding each other's unique needs, identifying where shared needs lie, and developing more specific demands to meet all communities' needs.[17–20] For example, individual ethnic community needs that emerged through focused research during the COVID-19 pandemic supported coalition-based advocacy for language access and health care for all.[21] CACF, working closely with advocates from across the country, developed explainers for advocates that reframe the zero–sum concern fed by a scarcity mindset as a unifying vision of solidarity.[22]

Bearing Context in Mind

CACF had to address concerns in AA and NH/PI communities rooted in fears based on the history of US anti-Asian policy. At a time of increasing racial acrimony and anti-immigrant sentiment, any policy change related to data collection raises concerns about data privacy and security. An ongoing challenge in this work is establishing trust between community members and government agencies tasked with collecting their data.

Given the US history of promoting anti-Asian policies such as the Chinese Exclusion Act of 1882, the forced incarceration of Japanese Americans in World War II, and the post-9/11 surveillance and persecution of South Asian, Indo-Caribbean, Middle Eastern, and North African Americans, any data collection practice must include ample guardrails to ensure data privacy and security while balancing the need for more publicly available comprehensive data.[16,17] Framing data as the foundation of public policy and framing complete and accurate data as a civil rights issue helped make it more accessible and relevant to community audiences, which is especially critical to the public health response during a pandemic.[22]

Visibility for Small Populations

Another obstacle to data disaggregation is the perception that AA and NH/PI populations are separately too small to be statistically significant. Many established institutions analyzing demographic trends include White, Black, and Hispanic/Latino but exclude or otherize Asian and NH/PI by lumping them into the catchall of Other. Populations with samples that are traditionally thought to be small often struggle in silence and require attention from public health researchers.[5]

Strategies for oversampling certain populations or for employing standardized and detailed race and ethnicity categories that may be combined with data from multiple surveys can facilitate inquiry into the health and social service needs of small populations.[1] Because AA and NH/PI populations are small but growing, disaggregation practices must contemplate ways to identify small populations and maximize the possibility of collecting data consistently across agencies and levels of government while balancing privacy concerns.[1,3]

Working in Coalition

Successful advocacy for these changes requires a diverse set of stakeholders (e.g., legislators, government agency officials, and media) and, especially, community leadership from the populations whose data are collected. Strong bidirectional communication about the concerns of the communities that will be affected by changes to data are essential. Tensions or gaps in trust must be bridged as this work advances. AA and NH/PI–serving community-based organizations were the core members of the INM coalition. At critical times, especially during the height of the legislative season, INM met at least monthly and sometimes more often with a steering committee of approximately 15 to 20 AA and NH/PI–serving community-based organizations.

Community-based organizations are directly affected by the lack of disaggregated data. They depend on city, state, and federal data collection to reflect the needs of underserved communities to drive adequate resources and appropriate policies that can meet those needs. INM stakeholders and allies include elected officials, government agency personnel, researchers and academics, media, health advocates, and, most importantly, community members who wish to be represented in government data collection.[23]

CACF was successful also because it worked with other populations invested in data equity, including advocates from the LGBTQ+ (lesbian, gay, bisexual, transgender/-sexual, queer or questioning, and all subsects) community interested in sexual orientation and gender identity data disaggregation. The need for disaggregated data and reform of government data collection practices are shared by Black, White, Latino, Middle Eastern and North African, American Indian, Alaska Native, immigrant, and LGBTQ+ communities. Each type of stakeholder brings a unique set of skills, best practices, perspective, power, network, and political influence to the campaign.

Building Relationships With Champions

Over many years, INM's relationships with New York City and New York State legislators enabled them to see progress on both city and state laws. Councilmember Daniel Dromm's proposal to package data disaggregation based on ancestry, languages spoken, multiracial identity, and sexual orientation and gender identity led to the successful passage of three combined laws.[24] At the state level, advocates worked with Assembly Member Yuh-Line Niou (D) and Senator Julia Salazar (D) to build consistent support for disaggregation by framing it as a question of efficiency, asking legislators how they could hold agencies accountable for efficiently deploying resources if they did not understand the existing needs. The bill passed both houses in 2019 but was vetoed by then-governor Cuomo.

In the wake of increased anti-Asian violence in 2020 and 2021, CACF redoubled efforts to draw attention to the root causes of violence and elevated data equity as a critical component of addressing health, wellness, and safety for AA and NH/PI communities. With a mobilizing letter to Governor Cuomo in 2021, INM cultivated broad-based support for AA and NH/PI data disaggregation among legislators, especially those whose constituents included a significant proportion of AA and NH/PI. INM sought bipartisan supporters, many of whom responded to arguments for the cost-saving efficiency of government systems: 2 Republican assembly members sponsored the bill, and half of all Republican senators voted to pass the law.

In December 2021, New York State enacted a historic state data disaggregation law that was signed by Governor Kathy Hochul (D). This win laid the groundwork for follow-up successes. In 2023, the New York State Senate also passed S.6584, which, if enacted, will mandate the disaggregation for Middle Eastern and North African populations, who up until now have been categorized as White.[25]

Securing Government Implementation Funding

Data equity and meaningful disaggregation require system-level changes to the governmental agency data systems. These changes require government investment for successful implementation. Changing laws without an accompanying budget allocation to support infrastructure improvements across government agencies may lead to inaccurate data or challenges in implementation. Although it may be costly to implement better data infrastructure and capacity, communities that are not recognized, and in turn society, pay for data gaps and invisibility every day.

Ensuring Implementation

The nuts and bolts of disaggregation advocacy happen not only when the bill is written and signed into law, or only when a regulation is adopted, but also when it is implemented by a government agency. Without the effective and equitable implementation of data disaggregation, systems risk sharing and using inaccurate or biased data of communities that are assumed to be truthful.

Recognizing the importance of a community-informed process to ensure accurate implementation of data disaggregation laws, once the city law was passed, INM engaged with city agency officials to support the work to disaggregate city data. Improving data quality and descriptiveness requires transparency, dialogue, and relationship building among service providers, government officials, and researchers to be able to ascertain the processes of disaggregating data, including collection and information sharing with the community.

INM sought administrators familiar with data collection, infrastructure, and equity-related policies and processes in agencies and asked questions such as, What language is the data collected in? How are government systems training staff to collect the data? Who is involved in survey creation? How is the community involved in efforts to collect and disseminate their data? When are data being collected? Is data collection tied to existing forms or a voluntary form (which may elicit different responses from individuals than a required one)? It was important for advocates to understand the internal technical, financial, and political obstacles that might slow government agencies' implementation of data disaggregation. Understanding the challenges of unfunded mandates and establishing consistency across varying jurisdictions help to establish trust and lead to better advocacy.

CHALLENGES AND OPPORTUNITIES AHEAD

Resistance can act as a drag on the momentum needed to secure resources, build national partnerships, and win policy changes for data disaggregation. The notion that these efforts lack meaningful support can become a self-fulfilling prophecy, impeding local and state efforts for better data. Progress in New York serves as a model to activate comparable campaigns for data disaggregation as part of broader efforts for data equity.

CACF is already building on its initial successes by being part of a data disaggregation network that was developed and assembled by The Leadership Conference Education Fund, in which groups share their knowledge and experiences and work with other state and local groups to foster change from the community level to the national level. As public health seeks to be at the forefront of efforts for data equity, centering the fight for disaggregated data for all populations is essential. Winning descriptive and illuminating data are possible with tenacity, relationships, and by working in coalition. AJPH

CORRESPONDENCE

Correspondence should be sent to Claudia M. Calhoon, Department of Health and Human Performance, CUNY York College, 94-20 Guy R Brewer Blvd, Jamaica, NY 11451 (e-mail: ccalhoon@york.cuny.edu). Reprints can be ordered at http://www.ajph.org by clicking the "Reprints" link.

PUBLICATION INFORMATION

Full Citation: Gundanna A, Calhoon CM, Anand M, Feng L, Leung V. Championing the 2021 New York State law: a step toward data disaggregation on Asian Americans, Native Hawaiians, and Pacific Islanders. *Am J Public Health*. 2023;113(12): 1296–1300.

Acceptance Date: August 19, 2023.

DOI: https://doi.org/10.2105/AJPH.2023.307428

CONTRIBUTORS

A. Gundanna, C. M. Calhoon, and L. Feng drafted portions of the article and contributed to subsequent revisions. M. Anand and V. Leung provided content expertise related to data disaggregation and the national context of data equity and contributed to substantial revisions. All authors made substantial contributions to the conceptualization, design, and content of the article.

ACKNOWLEDGMENTS

We thank Patrick McNeil for reading a draft of the article. The authors acknowledge with deep gratitude the Asian American, Native Hawaiian, and Pacific Islander communities working in continued advocacy for data equity through data disaggregation.

CONFLICTS OF INTEREST

The authors have no conflicts of interest to disclose.

REFERENCES

1. Islam N, Khan S, Kwon SC, Jang D, Ro M, Trinh-Shevrin C. Methodological issues in the collection, analysis, and reporting of granular data in Asian American populations: historical challenges

and potential solutions. *J Health Care Poor Underserved.* 2010;21(4):1354–1381. https://doi.org/10.1353/hpu.2010.0939

2. Kauh TJ, Read JG, Scheitler AJ. The critical role of racial/ethnic data disaggregation for health equity. *Popul Res Policy Rev.* 2021;40(1):1–7. https://doi.org/10.1007/s11113-020-09631-6
3. Shimkhada R, Scheitler AJ, Ponce NA. Capturing racial/ethnic diversity in population-based surveys: data disaggregation of health data for Asian American, Native Hawaiian, and Pacific Islanders (AANHPIs). *Popul Res Policy Rev.* 2021;40:81–102. https://doi.org/10.1007/s11113-020-09634-3
4. Teranishi RT, Nguyen BMD, Alcantar CM. The Asian American and Pacific Islander data disaggregation movement: the convergence of community activism and policy reform. *Asian American Policy Review.* 2014;25:26–36.
5. Lee M, Sumibcay JRC, Cory H, Duarte C, Planey AM. Extending critical race, racialization, and racism literatures to the adoption, implementation, and sustainability of data equity policies and data (dis)aggregation practices in health research. *Health Serv Res.* 2023;58(suppl 2):262–267. https://doi.org/10.1111/1475-6773.14167
6. Srinivasan S, Guillermo T. Toward improved health: disaggregating Asian American and Native Hawaiian/Pacific Islander data. *Am J Public Health.* 2000;90(11):1731–1734. https://doi.org/10.2105/AJPH.90.11.1731
7. Budiman A, Ruiz NG. Asian Americans are the fastest-growing racial or ethnic group in the US April 9, 2021. Available at: https://www.pewresearch.org/short-reads/2021/04/09/asian-americans-are-the-fastest-growing-racial-or-ethnic-group-in-the-u-s. Accessed June 20, 2023.
8. Frey WH. Mapping America's diversity with the 2020 census. September 21, 2021. Available at: https://www.brookings.edu/research/mapping-americas-diversity-with-the-2020-census. Accessed June 20, 2023.
9. US Census Bureau. Asian alone or in any combination by selected groups. 2021. Available at: https://data.census.gov/table?q=asian+groups&tid=ACSDT1Y2021.B02018. Accessed July 7, 2023.
10. Edlagan C, Vaghul K. How data disaggregation matters for Asian Americans and Pacific Islanders. December 14, 2016. Available at: https://equitablegrowth.org/how-data-disaggregation-matters-for-asian-americans-and-pacific-islanders. Accessed June 20, 2023.
11. Chin MK, Đoàn LN, Yi SS, Wong JA, Kwon SC. Asian-American COVID-19 experience. February 23, 2021. Available at: https://med.nyu.edu/departments-institutes/population-health/divisions-sections-centers/health-behavior/sites/default/files/pdf/csaah-asian-american-covid19-experience.pdf. Accessed June 20, 2023.
12. Kalyanaraman Marcello R, Dolle J, Tariq A, et al. Disaggregating Asian race reveals COVID-19 disparities among Asian American patients at New York City's public hospital system. *Public Health Rep.* 2022;137(2):317–325. https://doi.org/10.1177/00333549211061313
13. Ahébée S. "Without data, there's no equity": Deficient Asian American COVID-19 data masked community-wide disparities. March 14, 2021. Available at: https://whyy.org/articles/without-data-theres-no-equity-deficient-asian-american-covid-19-data-masked-community-wide-disparities. Accessed June 28, 2023.
14. AA & NH/PI Health Central. NYC COVID-19 community resources and needs assessment. 2022. Available at: https://aanhpihealth.org/resource/nyc-covid-19-community-resources-and-needs-assessment-nyc-covid-19-chrna. Accessed June 28, 2023.
15. Wang SC, Santos BMC. At the intersection of the model minority myth and antiblackness: from Asian American triangulation to recommendations for solidarity. *J Couns Psychol.* 2023;70(4):352–366. https://doi.org/10.1037/cou0000662
16. Kader F, Đoàn LN, Lee M, Chin MK, Kwon SC, Yi SS. Disaggregating race/ethnicity data categories: criticisms, dangers, and opposing viewpoints. *Health Affairs Forefront.* March 25, 2022. https://doi.org/10.1377/forefront.20220323.555023
17. Aguirre A, Lio S. Spaces of mobilization: the Asian American/Pacific Islander struggle for social justice. *Soc Justice.* 2008;35(2):1–17. Available at: https://www.proquest.com/docview/231929778/abstract/B6CAB4D4536F4AC9PQ/1. Accessed July 11, 2023.
18. Gundanna A. Collective identity and identity work in a nonprofit organizational coalition. 2018. Available at: https://www.proquest.com/openview/5268c370eaca13d91acca33b0aaf59ae/1/advanced. Accessed July 11, 2023.
19. Umemoto K. "On Strike!" San Francisco State College strike, 1968–69: the role of Asian American students. *Amerasia J.* 1989;15:1, 3–41. https://doi.org/10.17953/amer.15.1.7213030j5644rx25
20. Coalition for Asian American Children and Families. Who we are: Asian Americans in NY. 2022. Available at: https://www.youtube.com/watch?v=ByPO2wY6Tw4. Accessed July 10, 2023.
21. Coalition for Asian American Children and Families. What is data disaggregation? Available at: https://www.facebook.com/photo/?fbid=619311226906948&set=a.415554330615973. Accessed August 15, 2023.
22. Coalition for Asian American Children and Families. Frequently asked questions on NYS law S7821/A8743: AA and NH/PI data disaggregation. Available at: https://docs.google.com/document/d/1r8TyFMN3Z6MaalFiXiGrohb7ahciKypU9CQRbdo7AcY/edit?usp=embed_facebook. Accessed July 10, 2023.
23. Coalition for Asian American Children and Families. What is data disaggregation? An explainer. January 19, 2022. Available at: https://www.facebook.com/photo/?fbid=10158730372896485&set=pcb.10158730380036485. Accessed August 15, 2023.
24. City of New York. Local law no. 126. 2016. Available at: https://nyc.legistar1.com/nyc/attachments/f959cc8b-4700-437b-b1a7-675805361cc4.pdf. Accessed June 21, 2023.
25. Gianaris M. Senate deputy leader Gianaris announces senate unanimously passes widely-supported legislation expanding recognition of Middle Eastern, North African individuals in state data. June 9, 2023. Available at: https://www.nysenate.gov/newsroom/press-releases/2023/michael-gianaris/senate-deputy-leader-gianaris-announces-senate. Accessed June 21, 2023.

Social Determinants of Health, Quality of Public Health Data, and Health Equity in the United States

Steven H. Sheingold, PhD, Rachael B. Zuckerman, PhD, Nancy De Lew, MA, and Andre Chappel, PhD

See also Toward More Equitable Public Health Data, pp. 1276–1300.

In recent years, increasing attention has been paid to the impact social determinants of health (SDOH) can have on health equity in the United States.

In this essay, we provide a framework for considering the upstream structural factors that affect the distribution of SDOH as well as the downstream consequences for individuals and groups. Improving health equity in the United States will require multiple policy streams, each requiring comprehensive data for policy development, implementation, and evaluation.

Although much progress has been made in improving these data, there remain considerable gaps and opportunities for improvement. (*Am J Public Health*. 2023;113(12):1301–1308. https://doi.org/10.2105/AJPH.2023.307423)

AJPH December 2023, Vol 113, No. 12

In recent years, increasing attention has been paid to the impact social determinants of health (SDOH) can have on health equity in the United States. Yet improving health equity in the United States will require comprehensive data for policy development, implementation, and evaluation. Although much progress has been made in improving these data, there remain considerable gaps and opportunities for improvement.

The recent COVID-19 pandemic exposed and exacerbated many inequities in our society, including those affecting health outcomes. American Indian or Alaska Native, Black, and Hispanic or Latino people experienced greater rates of infection, hospitalization, and death from the virus than did White people.[1,2] Although it is important to have real-time data that are sufficient to formulate and implement policies responsive to the needs of all populations during public health emergencies, it is critical to realize that these disparate effects of COVID-19 are symptomatic of long-standing health inequities in our system. To address underlying systemic drivers of such health inequities, there is an ongoing need for high-quality, timely data that extends beyond the recent pandemic.

Addressing SDOH is a component of the Biden–Harris Administration's larger health equity agenda. As defined in Executive Order 13985, the term "equity" means the consistent and systematic fair, just, and impartial treatment of all individuals, including individuals who belong to underserved communities that have been denied such treatment, such as Black, Latino, Indigenous and Native American persons, Asian Americans, Native Hawaiians, Pacific Islanders, and other persons of color; members of religious minorities; lesbian, gay, bisexual, transgender, and queer persons; persons with disabilities; persons who live in rural areas; and persons otherwise adversely affected by persistent poverty or inequality.[3] According to the Centers for Disease Control and Prevention (CDC), health equity is achieved when every person has the opportunity to "attain his or her full health potential" and no one is "disadvantaged from achieving this potential because of social position or other socially determined circumstances."[4]

In this essay, we argue that several types of data are needed to inform and support policies to address SDOH, their upstream structural causes, their downstream consequences for individuals and groups, and their interrelationships with the medical care system. We first present a conceptual framework to describe the relationships SDOH have with health equity as a guide to data needs. We then discuss currently available data and the gaps that exist in fulfilling these needs.

CONCEPTUAL FRAMEWORK

The Office of the Assistant Secretary for Planning and Evaluation (ASPE) has developed a conceptual framework (abbreviated framework in Figure 1; detailed framework in Figure A; available as a supplement to the online version of this article at http://www.ajph.org) to guide ASPE's work on health equity. This framework can help in considering potential policy solutions and assessing knowledge and evidence gaps. It is not, however, a fully predictive model of how key drivers affect specific disparities in outcomes. It recognizes that health equity can be assessed by examining disparities in health indicators (e.g., life expectancy, active life expectancy) and assessing the medical and social drivers of these disparities. These drivers include broad, interrelated aspects of the social, legal, and institutional environment affecting communities such as structural discrimination, physical environment, employment, income and wealth, education, and access to high-quality health care. Most importantly, it is a framework for thinking about the multiple and interrelated social and medical care drivers of health so they can be addressed more comprehensively in policy development and data needs.

The framework is described in detail elsewhere[5]; here, we highlight the parts most relevant to the current discussion of data needs. The first critical aspect—identified in the "Populations Negatively Affected by SDOH" bar at the top of Figure 1—is the groups for which concerns about disparities in outcomes, opportunity, and experience arise. Assessing equity requires making comparisons between groups with different levels of social advantage.[6] In virtually every society, social advantage—and its corresponding position in social hierarchies—varies according to socioeconomic, racial, ethnic, gender, age, and geographic differences. In addition, various forms of discrimination can play a significant role in disadvantaging some groups.[7]

The rest of Figure 1 illustrates various nonmedical and medical individual and systemic drivers that combine to influence disparities in outcomes observed (example in Box D1 in Figure 1). These drivers are shown in the 3 columns of the figure: (1) nonmedical determinants, (2) access to care, and (3) experience in the medical care system. The top and middle rows, moving from left to right, provide examples of inequities that affect health. The middle row provides examples of the structural factors affecting health equity, and the top row reflects how these factors are experienced by individuals and communities. The bottom row provides examples of policies that can affect the drivers and outcomes in rows 1 and 2. Box D2 displays examples of health-related social needs (HRSNs), which are distinct from SDOH but must be addressed along

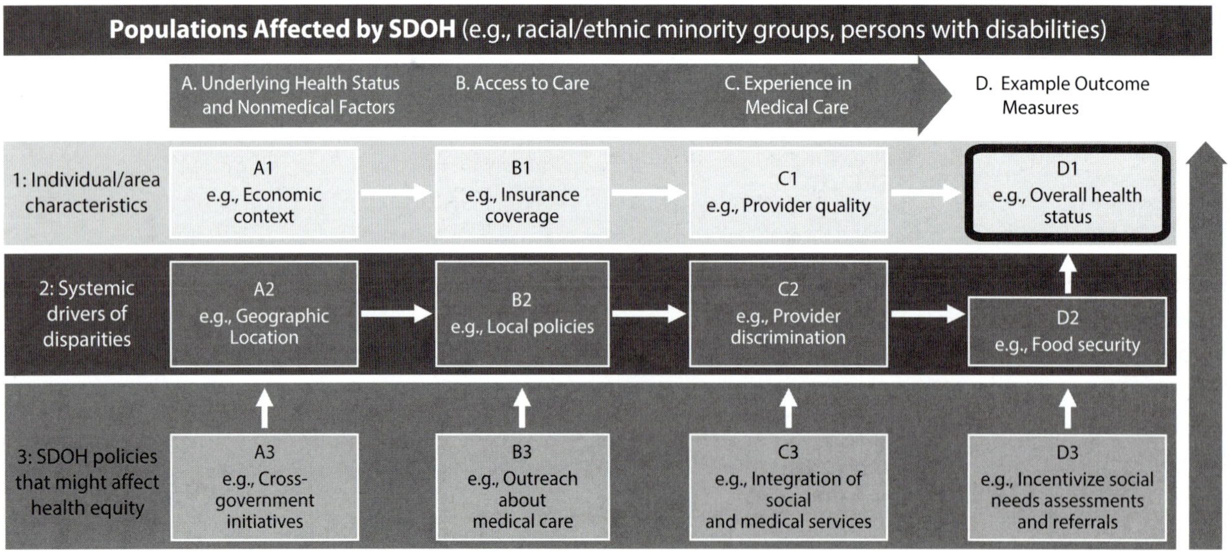

FIGURE 1— A Conceptual Framework for Addressing Social Determinants of Health (SDOH)

Note. For a full version of this framework, see Figure A, available as a supplement to the online version of this article at https://www.ajph.org.

with medical care to improve health outcomes.

POLICY STRATEGIES AND DATA NEEDS

A comprehensive approach to addressing SDOH to improve health equity requires strategies across all levels of government that we group into 5 categories:

1. Address individual-level HRSNs in communities by using incentives for medical care providers to screen for HRSNs and refer to appropriate services and community assistance to ensure that these services are available.
2. Address the underlying systemic determinants (e.g., structural discrimination) that affect the distribution of HRSNs, SDOH, access to care, and quality of care.
3. Improve the distribution of community-level SDOH using whole-of-government approaches for improving economic activities, environment, housing, food availability, transportation, and so on.
4. Bolster access to health care by expanding insurance coverage and the supply of services and facilities in currently underserved areas.
5. Advance quality of care by reducing disparities in care, increasing the provision of culturally and linguistically appropriate care and services to reduce discrimination in care, and ensuring that members of historically underserved communities have training opportunities so the future workforce will reflect the populations served.

Developing, implementing, and evaluating policies in these 5 categories will be challenging across governments at all levels and their community partners. These efforts will require improvements in public health data to identify factors driving observed disparities and how they can best be addressed via the 5 policy categories.

From a national policy perspective, data standardized across programs and data systems allow comparison and data sharing across programs, similar to current hospital discharge data and vital records. But most importantly, the data must contain elements to identify disparities between groups and to analyze the factors contributing to such disparities and the impact of policy interventions intended to address them. Arguably, current data allow researchers and policymakers to assess measures of access and quality of care (categories 4 and 5) more thoroughly than the other categories. Thus, for the remainder of the essay we focus on data for structural discrimination, SDOH, and HRSNs to support the other policy categories.

CURRENT STATUS, GAPS, AND INITIATIVES

Based on the conceptual framework described, a complete set of SDOH-related data would include elements that are not widely available in public health data at this time and are developed with communities. These include data to identify disparities in health outcomes and the social drivers (SDOH, HRSNs, and structural factors) of these disparities.

In this essay, we take a broad view in defining public health data. Specifically, we focus on resources from within and outside public health for the purpose of measuring and improving public health and health equity. Under this broader view, public health data can come from a variety of sources, including surveys, insurance claims, surveillance data, disease registries, vital records, medical records, environmental pollution, water quality, built environment, community vaccination rates, education, employment, justice system involvement, and more. Public health data can include both individual-level and aggregated data. These data sources vary in terms of availability, quality, and interoperability for populations affected, as well as their appropriateness for specific types of public health and policy uses.

Data to Identify Affected Populations

Although some of the groups of concern identified in the executive order are more often captured in public health data, others are rarely included. For example, some databases that contribute to public health data, such as public health surveillance systems, include race and ethnicity information. Other data sources that could be helpful do not, such as private insurance claims for research.[8] Although race and ethnicity are often collected, most data sources do not include information to identify sexual orientation and gender identity or disability status. For example, Centers for Medicare & Medicaid Services (CMS) programs (Medicare, Medicaid, and the Federally Facilitated Marketplace) do not collect such data in any standardized format, although a few states do collect these data in their Medicaid programs.[9]

Even in cases in which equity data are collected, there may be limitations. For example, despite the existence of race and ethnicity fields in many data sources, there are differing definitions of race/ethnicity, varying levels of detail, challenges with missing data, and unresolved questions about the accuracy for particular groups among these data sources. Moreover, studies using race/ethnicity data often lack the methodological details needed to assess their validity and replicate results.[10] Other gaps include when such data are intentionally not collected or reported to protect patient privacy, particularly when data are collected on a small number of individuals or when there may be heightened sensitivities about potential repercussions for individuals because of the nature of the data. Efforts to address these health equity–related data uses are already under way. For example, CMS is pursuing its future vision for health equity data, including, where applicable and appropriate, alignment with the Department of Health and Human Services' United States Core Data for Interoperability overseen by the Office of the National Coordinator for Health Information Technology. Additionally, the Office of Management and Budget has proposed to update the federal government's race and ethnicity data standards.[11]

There are existing data sources that could start to fill these gaps as well. Claims from public and private insurers are a staple of health services research and have the potential to greatly improve the availability of individual-level data for addressing health equity issues. These data have many advantages, including large sample sizes and patient-level information, that can be used for studying costs, utilization, practice patterns, burden of illness, and access and quality issues, as well as for forming the basis for policy simulations. Eventually, these data may include information on patients' HRSNs. There are also well-known gaps and issues with claims data that can limit the scope and usefulness of some research efforts, particularly with regard to addressing health equity. Among these gaps are the exclusion of information not needed for reimbursement, including equity information such as race and ethnicity, and the proprietary nature of many claims databases requiring analyses at higher aggregation levels and preventing the comparison of claims across payers to understand the full population.[12]

Structural Factors

For the purposes of developing data and policy, it is important to distinguish between SDOH and HRSNs. SDOH affect everyone; they are not something an individual can have or not have, and they are not inherently positive or negative.[13] Whether they contribute to either positive or negative community- and individual-level outcomes depends on the nature of the SDOH in a community. The policy levers to address SDOH also exist above the individual level, at the community level or other geographic area. For instance, a community may have an insufficient supply of affordable housing as well as unequal distribution of such housing that may result in high levels of housing instability for some residents of the community. Policies to address the community's supply of affordable housing require community-level interventions, such as designating that a certain portion of new housing be affordable.

Although SDOH exist at a community or other geographic level, HRSNs describe an individual's experience. For example, individuals' inability to access nutritious food and maintain a healthy diet may be related to their community being a "food desert," that is, lacking in accessible supermarkets or farmers markets. To best support policy development and implementation, it is important to distinguish between SDOH and HRSNs, particularly with regard to the data that are needed.

To assist health care providers in helping to address HRSNs, there have been suggestions to use area-level deprivation indices to adjust Medicare and Medicaid payments.[14] Existing measures of area deprivation have been found to be weakly correlated with HRSNs.[15,16] In practice, a particular community may lack abundant affordable housing, but a single individual in the area may have stable housing, whereas another may experience homelessness, resulting in only the second person having a HRSN. Policies to address HRSNs include having medical care providers screen patients for these needs and refer them to appropriate community-level services and assisting communities to develop platforms for such referrals and ensure the availability of these services.

As policy discussions focus on SDOH and health equity, additional attention has been paid to the structural factors in our systems that result in health disparities; that is, individuals with particular characteristics may be subject to structural inequities that produce adverse health outcomes.[17] A particular focus has been placed on structural racism, which can be defined as the macrolevel systems, social forces, institutions, ideologies, and processes that interact with one another to generate and reinforce inequities among racial and ethnic groups.[18] Structural racism leads to "differential access to the goods, services, and opportunities of society by race,"[19(p1212)] determines societal values and power structures, and underlies persistent health disparities in the United States.[20] We use the term "structural discrimination" because factors that result in unequal distributions of SDOH and HRSNs and unequal access to high-quality medical care, all of which contribute to poor health outcomes, affect other groups as well (e.g. rural residents). Structural discrimination is different from individual experiences of discrimination, which happen to an individual, rather than a society. But both types of discrimination are harmful to health equity.

Each individual in their community has a unique combination of HRSN, SDOH, and structural discrimination, and their experiences and needs exist at the intersection of these. To truly address social drivers of health, data and policies need to capture not only the group differences but the intersectional impacts as well.

Although we use these concepts distinctly in this essay, in other cases they have all been referred to as SDOH or social risk factors. Here, we will use language based on the definitions we have discussed although source material may use another term.

Health-Related Social Needs Data

Much progress has been made in collecting HRSN data over the past few years. In a 2020 report to Congress, ASPE discussed the then current state of HRSN data collection.[21] At that time, more than one third of Medicaid managed care plans had reported collecting or planning to collect data on HRSNs in the 2018 to 2019 plan year; the Centers for Medicare and Medicaid Innovation was requiring entities participating in the accountable health communities model to use the CMS-developed HRSNs screening tool (although many other tools were being used in the health care system); and health care providers were beginning to use *International Classification of Disease, 10th Revision* (*ICD-10*) Z codes to identify HRSNs in health care claims. Today, all of these efforts have been expanded, and new efforts to improve HRSNs data have begun.

One of the major obstacles to improving HRSNs data collection that ASPE identified was the lack of incentives for health care providers to collect these data, and much has been done to address this. The Centers for Medicare and Medicaid Innovation is encouraging participants in all new payment models to collect HRSNs information though a validated screening tool.[9] Moreover, CMS has introduced hospital quality measures assessing the proportion of patients screened and the proportion that screen positive for HRSNs. Additionally, Medicare Advantage Special Needs Plans are required to screen enrollees for HRSNs as part of an annual risk assessment.[9] CMS has also increased providers' incentives to use *ICD-10* Z codes to identify HRSNs by including documented HRSNs in clinical severity and corresponding payment rates.[22,23]

Another challenge ASPE identified was the inability to share HRSNs data once collected, and much progress has been made in developing data collection and exchange standards to share HRSNs across the health and social service ecosystem. The Office of the National Coordinator for Health Information Technology has included HRSNs and health equity elements in the United States Core Data for Interoperability, version 2, potentially increasing the ease of exchanging this information across the health care system.[24] Over the past 4 years, the _Gravity Project has worked to "develop consensus-driven data standards to support the collection, use, and exchange of data" on HRSNs, creating value sets and use cases for a number of HRSNs that can now be more easily captured and exchanged.[25]

Despite this progress, many of the challenges ASPE identified have not yet been addressed. Although data sharing has become easier, there are still many different screening tools being used, so information may not be comparable across data sources. Additionally, even when validated screening tools are used, they may not be used consistently, resulting in undocumented HRSNs. This is evident from the still low use of Z codes in Medicare claims.[26] More work will need to be done to consistently screen for HRSNs in a way that allows comparison across data sets.

Social Determinants of Health Data

In practice, SDOH data tend to be operationalized as area-level measures of deprivation. The available SDOH data include resources available in a community and community-level characteristics of the population. Although some of these SDOH data have been available for decades, new efforts are making the information more readily accessible and aggregated in a single data set. For example, the Agency for Healthcare Research and Quality has aggregated much of this information into a SDOH database,[27] and the CDC has developed the PLACES (population-level analysis and community estimates) data set that combines small-area SDOH and health status information.[28]

Rather than measuring community-level resources (e.g., affordable housing stock or availability of public transport), much of the existing SDOH data come from survey responses that are aggregated to represent the social characteristics of the population in an area (e.g., proportion of homeless respondents or those with access to a private vehicle). Many CDC surveys include SDOH modules, such as the Behavioral Risk Factor Surveillance System, the Youth Risk Factor Surveillance System, and the Pregnancy Risk Assessment Monitoring System. In particular, Census' American Community Survey provides a rich data source for small-area measures and has been used to understand specific SDOH and to create multidimension SDOH indices that summarize an area's level of social deprivation, such as the Area Deprivation Index and the Social Vulnerability Index. However, the applicability of these indices for policy has come under scrutiny.[29] Additionally, not all SDOH domains are included in these indices; most include a measure of income or wealth, but population-level HRSNs are much less likely to be included in an index.[5] Furthermore, a report from the National Commission to Transform Public Health Data Systems found that many individual data sources capture only a few of the SDOH domains, making it difficult to understand the full SDOH picture using a single data source.[30] Additional work on these indices will make them more useful for policymakers.

In addition to the aggregate population characteristics, SDOH can be measured by the services and infrastructure of an area, such as the availability of public transportation, healthy food, health services, affordable housing, temperature, and environmental pollutants. Although these measures are available, as evidenced by their inclusion in the Agency for Healthcare Research and Quality SDOH database, they are not typically included in area-level SDOH indices. Thus, these indices are often missing an important component: they identify the population's needs but not the availability of services to address those needs.

Finally, some important SDOH are rarely, if ever, captured. For example, the National Commission to Transform Public Health Data Systems notes that the domains of community and civic well-being are generally missing from existing data,[29] limiting the ability of policies to account for these important community factors.

A challenge with SDOH data is understanding what the appropriate uses are for specific elements and how to use data to effectively target interventions. Although the availability and awareness of SDOH data are increasing, additional efforts are needed to determine which measures or indices are appropriate for different uses, so that programs and policymakers have guidance when selecting data sources. Additional information on the development of SDOH data elements, their applicability to specific populations, their validity at varying geographic levels (i.e., census block, zip code, county), and their association with outcomes of interest would make these decisions easier.

Data on Structural Factors

Across the 3 types of data, structural factors are often the hardest to measure. Regardless, measuring structural discrimination as a component of public health data needs attention, as this is an underlying factor that drives many of the disparities in SDOH, HRSNs, and health outcomes. To clearly demonstrate and understand the mechanisms that produce these differences in health outcomes and craft appropriate policies to address these disparities, we will need data that include direct measures of structural discrimination. For example, a recent study reviewed a number of efforts to develop measures of structural racism and associate them with outcomes, but the authors find that much work remains to be done to establish universally accepted measures of structural racism.[31]

CONCLUSIONS

There has been a longstanding recognition that addressing social drivers of health is critical to improving the nation's health.[32] In recent years, the policy debate has recognized the need to address social drivers of health both to improve the health status of all Americans and to address the issues that disadvantage some populations in achieving optimal health. The Biden–Harris Administration has made health equity a top priority and has begun a number of initiatives to improve access to and quality of care as well as address SDOH and HRSNs.

The objective of these efforts is to minimize disparities in key indicators of health status among groups by eliminating systematic differences in the drivers of health, such as SDOH and HRSNs. These efforts will require better data to develop, implement, and evaluate policies. As described in this essay, numerous data sources have emerged in recent years, but there are gaps and inconsistencies that may inhibit evidence-based policymaking. It is time to develop and disseminate key indicators of structural factors, SDOH, and HRSNs that are standardized, can identify key groups of interest, and are available nationally and at local levels. Developing these data would require resources as well as addressing important issues of statutory requirements, confidentiality, and proprietary concerns. Importantly, succeeding will require engaging communities to understand what data should be collected, from whom, and how. Although progress has been made in recent years, additional opportunities remain to use existing data and plan for ongoing data system improvements to support public health efforts to promote health equity. AJPH

ABOUT THE AUTHORS

All authors are with the Office of the Assistant Secretary for Planning and Evaluation, US Department of Health and Human Services, Washington, DC.

CORRESPONDENCE

Correspondence should be sent to Rachael Zuckerman, 200 Independence Ave SW, Washington, DC 20201 (e-mail: rachael.zuckerman@hhs.gov). Reprints can be ordered at http://www.ajph.org by clicking the "Reprints" link.

PUBLICATION INFORMATION

Full Citation: Sheingold SH, Zuckerman RB, De Lew N, Chappel A. Social determinants of health, quality of public health data, and health equity in the United States. *Am J Public Health*. 2023;113(12):1301–1308.

Acceptance Date: August 17, 2023.

DOI: https://doi.org/10.2105/AJPH.2023.307423

CONTRIBUTORS

S. H. Sheingold wrote the first draft of the essay. All authors contributed to the conceptualization, writing, review, and editing of the essay.

CONFLICTS OF INTEREST

There are no conflicts of interest to report.

HUMAN PARTICIPANT PROTECTION

No protocol approval was necessary because no human participants were involved in this study.

REFERENCES

1. Centers for Disease Control and Prevention. Risk for COVID-19 infection, hospitalization, and death by race/ethnicity. April 23, 2021. Available at: https://stacks.cdc.gov/view/cdc/105453. Accessed August 15, 2023.
2. Tarazi WW, Finegold K, Sheingold SH, Wong Samson L, Zuckerman R, Bosworth A. COVID-19–related deaths and excess deaths among Medicare fee-for-service beneficiaries. *Health Aff (Millwood)*. 2021;40(6):879–885. https://doi.org/10.1377/hlthaff.2020.02521
3. White House. Executive Order 13985. Executive order on advancing racial equity and support for underserved communities through the federal government. January 20, 2021. Available at: https://www.whitehouse.gov/briefing-room/presidential-actions/2021/01/20/executive-order-advancing-racial-equity-and-support-for-underserved-communities-through-the-federal-government. Accessed July 12, 2023.
4. Centers for Disease Control and Prevention. Advancing Health Equity in Chronic Disease Prevention and Management. December 8, 2022. Available at: https://www.cdc.gov/chronicdisease/healthequity/index.htm. Accessed July 12, 2023.
5. Sheingold S, Zuckerman R, Alberto C, Samson L, Lee E, Aysola V. Reflections accompanying a report on addressing social drivers of health: evaluating area-level indices. 2022. ASPE Pub. no. HP-2022-26. Available at: https://www.aspe.hhs.gov/sites/default/files/documents/7899f865d60f7bebf44d96bd3d6227ea/Area-level-Indices-ASPE-Reflections.pdf?_ga=2.260927629.1252443683.1687699108-1057308064.1683893124. Accessed July 12, 2023.
6. Braveman P, Gruskin S. Defining equity in health. *J Epidemiol Community Health*. 2003;57(4):254–258. https://doi.org/10.1136/jech.57.4.254
7. Agency for Healthcare Research and Quality. 2022 National healthcare quality and disparities report. AHRQ Pub. No. 22(23)-0030. Available at: https://www.ahrq.gov/sites/default/files/wysiwyg/research/findings/nhqrdr/2022qdr-final-es.pdf. Accessed July 12, 2023.
8. Zuckerman R, Grigorescu V, Sheingold S. Claims and provider payment data gaps for responding to COVID-19: a framework for future strategies on improving access and use. Office of the Assistant Secretary for Planning and Evaluation.
9. Centers for Medicare & Medicaid Services. The path forward: improving data to advance health equity solutions. November 2022. Available at: https://www.cms.gov/files/document/path-forwardhe-data-paper.pdf. Accessed July 12, 2023.
10. Martinez RAM, Smith NR, Wilbur RE, Andrabi N, Goodwin AN, Zivich PN. Threats to equity: missing methodological details about race and ethnicity in health research. *Health Affairs Forefront*. March 13, 2023. Available at: https://www.healthaffairs.org/content/forefront/threats-equity-missing-methodological-details-race-and-ethnicity-health-research. Accessed September 17, 2023. https://doi.org/10.1377/forefront.20230310.613486
11. Office of Management and Budget. Initial proposals for updating OMB's race and ethnicity statistical standards. *Fed Regist*. 2023;88(18):5375–5384.
12. Zuckerman R, Grigorescu V, Sheingold S. *Claims and Provider Payment Data Gaps for Responding to COVID-19: A Framework for Future Strategies on Improving Access and Use*. Washington, DC: Office of the Assistant Secretary for Planning and Evaluation. In press.
13. Green K, Zook M. When talking about social determinants, precision matters. *Health Affairs Forefront*. October 29, 2019. Available at: https://www.healthaffairs.org/content/forefront/talking-social-determinants-precision-matters. Accessed September 17, 2023.
14. Phillips RL, Ostrovsky A, Gilfillan R, Price D, Bazemore AW. Accounting for social risks in Medicare and Medicaid payments. February 1, 2023. Available at: https://www.commonwealthfund.org/blog/2023/accounting-social-risks-medicare-and-medicaid-payments. Accessed August 14, 2023.
15. Powers BW, Figueroa JF, Canterberry M, et al. Association between community-level social risk and spending among Medicare beneficiaries: implications for social risk adjustment and health equity. *JAMA Health Forum*. 2023;4(3):e230266–e230266. https://doi.org/10.1001/jamahealthforum.2023.0266
16. Cottrell EK, Hendricks M, Dambrun K, et al. Comparison of community-level and patient-level social risk data in a network of community health centers. *JAMA Netw Open*. 2020;3(10):e2016852–e2016852. https://doi.org/10.1001/jamanetworkopen.2020.16852
17. Williams MV, Perez L, Siddiqi S, Qureshi N, Sousa J, Huttinger A. Building the evidence base for social determinants of health interventions. May 2021. Available at: https://aspe.hhs.gov/reports/building-evidence-base-social-determinants-health-interventions. Accessed July 12, 2023.
18. Gee GC, Ford CL. Structural racism and health inequities: old issues, new directions. *Du Bois Rev*. 2011;8(1):115–132. https://doi.org/10.1017/S1742058X11000130
19. Jones CP. Levels of racism: a theoretic framework and a gardener's tale. *Am J Public Health*. 2000;90(8):1212–1215. https://doi.org/10.2105/AJPH.90.8.1212
20. Churchwell K, Elkind MSV, Benjamin RM, et al. Call to action: structural racism as a fundamental driver of health disparities: a presidential advisory from the American Heart Association. *Circulation*. 2020;142(24):e454–e468. https://doi.org/10.1161/CIR.0000000000000936
21. Office of the Assistant Secretary for Planning and Evaluation. Second report to Congress on social risk and Medicare's value-based purchasing programs. June 28, 2020. Available at: https://aspe.hhs.gov/pdf-report/second-impact-report-to-congress. Accessed July 12, 2023.
22. Centers for Medicare & Medicaid Services. FY 2024 Hospital Inpatient Prospective Payment System (IPPS) and Long-Term Care Hospital Prospective Payment System (LTCH PPS) proposed rule—CMS-1785-P. April 10, 2023. Available at: https://www.cms.gov/newsroom/fact-sheets/fy-2024-hospital-inpatient-prospective-payment-system-ipps-and-long-term-care-hospital-prospective. Accessed July 12, 2023.
23. Robeznieks A. Social determinants of health and medical coding: what to know. May 13, 2022. Available at: https://www.ama-assn.org/practice-management/cpt/social-determinants-health-and-medical-coding-what-know. Accessed July 12, 2023.
24. Office of the National Coordinator for Health Information Technology. Social determinants of health. February 16, 2023. Available at: https://www.healthit.gov/health-equity/social-determinants-health. Accessed July 12, 2023.
25. Health Level Seven International. The Gravity Project. July 12, 2023. Available at: https://confluence.hl7.org/display/GRAV. Accessed July 12, 2023.
26. Saynisch P, Storfer-Isser A, Onstad K, et al. Utilization of Z codes for social determinants of health among a sample of Medicare advantage enrollees, 2017 and 2019. April 2022. Available at: https://www.cms.gov/files/document/data-highlight-april-2022.pdf. Accessed July 12, 2023.
27. Agency for Healthcare Research and Quality. Social determinants of health database. June 2023.

Available at: https://www.ahrq.gov/sdoh/data-analytics/sdoh-data.html. Accessed July 12, 2023.

28. Centers for Disease Control and Prevention. About PLACES. October 18, 2021. Available at: https://www.cdc.gov/places/about/index.html. Accessed July 12, 2023.
29. Azar KMJ, Alexander M, Smits K, Tio A, deGhetaldi L. ACO benchmarks based on area deprivation index mask inequities. *Health Affairs Forefront*. February 17, 2023. Available at: https://www.healthaffairs.org/content/forefront/aco-benchmarks-based-area-deprivation-index-mask-inequities. Accessed September 17, 2023. https://doi.org/10.1377/forefront.20230215.8850
30. Christopher GC, Zimmerman EB, Chandra A, Martin LC, eds. Charting a course for an equity-centered data system: recommendations from the National Commission to Transform Public Health Data Systems. October 2021. Available at: https://www.nationalcollaborative.org/wp-content/uploads/2021/10/RWJF-Transforming-Public-Health-Data-Systems.pdf. Accessed July 12, 2023.
31. Groos M, Wallace ME, Hardeman RR, Theall KP. Measuring inequity: a systematic review of methods used to quantify structural racism. *J Health Dispar Res Pract*. 2018;11(2):13. Available at: https://digitalscholarship.unlv.edu/jhdrp/vol11/iss2/13. Accessed July 12, 2023.
32. Lurie N. What the federal government can do about the nonmedical determinants of health. *Health Aff (Millwood)*. 2002;21(2):94–106. https://doi.org/10.1377/hlthaff.21.2.94

Association Between the New York SAFE Act and Firearm Suicide and Homicide: An Analysis of Synthetic Controls, New York State, 1999–2019

Ibraheem M. Karaye, MD, DrPH, Gaia Knight, BS, and Corinne Kyriacou, MPH, PhD

See also Blais, p. 1238.

Objectives. To assess the association between the New York Secure Ammunition and Firearms Enforcement Act (NY SAFE Act) and firearm suicide and homicide rates.

Methods. We employed a synthetic controls approach to investigate the impact of the NY SAFE Act on firearm suicide and firearm homicide rates. We collected state-level data on firearm mortality from the Centers for Disease Control and Prevention's Wide-ranging Online Data for Epidemiologic Research (WONDER) database for the period 1999–2019. We derived statistical inference by using a permutation-based in-place placebo test.

Results. The implementation of the NY SAFE Act was associated with a significant reduction in firearm homicide rates, demonstrating a decrease of 63%. This decrease corresponds to an estimated prevention of 1697 deaths between 2013 and 2019. However, there was no association between the NY SAFE Act and firearm suicide rates.

Conclusions. As the responsibility for enacting firearm policies increasingly falls on states instead of the federal government, this study provides valuable information that can assist states in making evidence-based decisions regarding the development and implementation of firearm policies that prioritize public safety and aim to prevent firearm-related fatalities. (*Am J Public Health*. 2023;113(12):1309–1317. https://doi.org/10.2105/AJPH.2023.307400)

AJPH December 2023, Vol 113, No. 12

In 2022, the Supreme Court of the United States blocked a 111-year-old gun law that prohibited New York State residents from carrying concealed guns in public.[1] The Court ruled that the law was unconstitutional and violated residents' rights in the Second and Fourteenth Amendments.[1] Loosening gun laws has been found to be linked to an increase in homicides from firearms.[2–4] Firearm violence is a preventable public health crisis and a leading cause of premature death in New York and the United States.[5,6] Therefore, preventing firearm-related deaths, disabilities, and injuries warrants an empirical investigation of policies that are effective in protecting the public's health.

Firearm injuries account for 5.3 deaths per 100 000 New York population, which equates to 1052 deaths in 2020 alone.[7,8] On average, 1991 persons are injured by guns every year in New York, ranking the state 42nd in firearm injuries nationwide.[9] Although New York is the fourth-lowest in gun deaths nationally, the mortality rate from guns increased by 7% from 2011 to 2020, which is equivalent to an absolute increase of 55 more deaths during the past decade.[9] Firearm violence is also a cause of economic burden to New York, with $11.4 billion expended annually, including $301.2 million that is being subsidized by taxpayers.[9]

To limit gun-associated harm, several states, including New York, have enacted laws to regulate firearms.[10] Examples include mandating licensing requirements beyond the standard set by the federal government, requiring background checks before the purchase of firearms and ammunition, prohibiting individuals that demonstrate signs of harm—to themselves or others—from purchasing a firearm (red flag laws), and mandating gun owners to make a reasonable effort at keeping firearms out of reach of children and other prohibited persons (safe storage laws).[4,10] State legislative efforts have been heterogeneous and have resulted in varied firearm-related outcomes.[10] But, overall, states with a comprehensive set of legislative actions have recorded reduced firearm-related injuries and deaths.[10–13] Legislative actions are also more likely to result in reduced morbidity and mortality if they restrict child access to firearms, implement systematic measures to limit the process of firearm acquisition, regulate the use of assault weapons and large-capacity magazines, and prohibit individuals who demonstrate a risk of harm—to self or others—from purchasing a firearm.[11,13–16] Conversely, stand-your-ground and right-to-carry laws have been associated with increased firearm morbidity and mortality.[17,18]

The New York Secure Ammunition and Firearms Enforcement Act (NY SAFE Act) was enacted in New York in January 2013.[19] Under this Act, owning a magazine that can hold more than 7 rounds of ammunition became illegal.[19] NY SAFE Act also mandates national background checks for private firearm purchases, expands the definition of illegal assault weapons to include rifles and shotguns with a thumbhole stock, requires a list of every firearm owned by an individual whenever a permit is renewed, establishes stronger penalties for illegal firearm use, requires safe storage of firearms from convicts of a felony or domestic violence, requires owners to report lost or stolen firearms or ammunitions within 24 hours, requires the recertification of handgun permits every 5 years, and amends the New York Mental Hygiene Law to require the reporting of patients at risk for inflicting significant harm to themselves or others, among other provisions.[19]

Despite the passage of a decade since its enactment, the impact of the NY SAFE Act on firearm deaths remains largely unexplored in the existing literature. Previous studies have primarily focused on specific aspects of the Act, including its implications for individuals with mental health issues or its constitutionality.[20–24] This study aims to fill this significant research gap by employing a novel quasi-experimental design, the synthetic control method (SCM), to examine the association between the NY SAFE Act and firearm mortality. SCM has garnered widespread recognition as a groundbreaking innovation in the evaluation literature and has been hailed as "the most important innovation in the policy evaluation literature in the last fifteen years."[25(p9)] Unlike conventional approaches, SCM utilizes a data-driven approach to construct synthetic controls that closely resemble the treatment state, thereby enhancing the internal validity of the findings.[25] The aim of the current study was to assess the relationship between the implementation of the NY SAFE Act and firearm suicide and homicide rates.

METHODS

We used a quasi-experimental design to examine the relationship between the implementation of the NY SAFE Act and counterfactual firearm mortality rates, specifically firearm suicide and homicide. The analysis involved estimating the counterfactual rates using data from weighted control states. The study period spanned from 1999 to 2019, with the preintervention period covering 1999 to 2012 and the postintervention period from 2013 to 2019. We excluded the year 2020 from our analysis because of the higher number of recorded firearm deaths in the United States during the COVID-19 pandemic.[26]

Outcome Measures

Our primary outcome measures included age-adjusted rates of overall firearm mortality, firearm suicide, and firearm homicide per 100 000 persons. Data on firearm deaths were obtained from the Centers for Disease Control and Prevention's Wide-ranging Online Data for Epidemiologic Research (WONDER) database. We abstracted the following variables using the following *International Classification of Diseases, 10th Revision* (Geneva, Switzerland: World Health Organization; 1992) codes: W2–W34, X72–X74, X93–X95, Y22–Y24, Y35.0, and U01.4. All rates were age-adjusted to the 2000 US standard population using the direct method.

Mortality rates were occasionally suppressed in WONDER for confidential reasons or because of low counts deemed unreliable.[27] To address missing values, multiple imputation was employed, replacing them with the average mortality rate for the respective state. States with complete missing values were excluded from the analysis.

Covariates

We derived state-level characteristics that could potentially confound the association between the NY SAFE Act and firearm mortality from national registries and included as covariates in the analysis. From the US Census Bureau,[28] we obtained the state-level proportion of residents who were aged younger than 18 years or aged 65 years or older; the proportion of females; proportion who were non-Hispanic White, non-Hispanic Black, Hispanic, American Indian/Alaska Native, and Asian/Pacific Islander; the proportion of residents that were high-school graduates or higher, and those with bachelor's degree or higher; and for the entire population, the median household income, the proportion living in poverty, and the proportion without health insurance aged younger than 65 years. From the US Bureau of Labor Statistics,[29] we obtained the unemployment rate for every state included in this study.

Statistical Analysis

We used SCM to estimate the counterfactual rates of overall firearm mortality, firearm suicide, and firearm homicide for the state of New York. SCM offers a valuable alternative to conventional evaluation approaches and effectively addresses significant limitations in the field of firearm policy research, including the challenges of finding comparable intervention and control groups and the sensitivity of findings to specific modeling choices.[30]

This innovative approach involved leveraging preintervention data on outcomes and relevant predictors to assign weights to control states in the donor pool.[30] The objective was to create a weighted combination of control states that closely resembled the intervention state during the preintervention period.[25,30] By carefully selecting the weights, certain states were excluded from the synthetic control analysis. The resulting weighted average of states provided an approximation of what the outcomes would have been in the posttreatment period had there been no intervention.[31,32]

To evaluate the impact of the NY SAFE Act on firearm mortality rates, we conducted a comparative analysis between the postintervention rates of New York and its synthetic control group from 2013 to 2019. This approach allowed us to assess the effectiveness of the intervention by examining the differences between the observed rates in New York and the counterfactual rates predicted by the synthetic control group.

The synthetic control method does not rely on traditional measures of uncertainty or statistical significance.[31–34] Therefore, to assess the likelihood of observing firearm suicide and homicide rate differences equal to or greater than those observed in New York attributable to chance alone, we employed permutation-based in-place placebo tests. These tests involved conducting the same analysis multiple times by randomly shuffling (permuting) the assignment of the intervention among control states.[31–34] The underlying premise is that in the absence of an actual intervention, no effect is expected, although random variation in the postintervention period could occur.[31–34] We calculated the root mean square prediction error (RMSPE) ratio (RMSPE posttreatment/pretreatment) and examined the *P* value below .10 as described by Abadie et al., Chrisinger, and Galiani et al.[32–34] We excluded states with a poor fit before the intervention, indicated by an RMSPE exceeding twice that of the intervention state, from the analyses.

To calculate the estimated number of firearm deaths prevented by the NY SAFE Act from 2013 to 2019, we multiplied the relative difference in rate between New York and its synthetic control by New York's population size each year, summing the values across those years.

We conducted all statistical analyses with Stata version 17.0 (StataCorp LP, College Station, TX).

Sensitivity Analysis

We assessed whether the implementation of the NY SAFE Act was associated with any potential substitution effect leading to increased deaths from nonfirearms. The results of this analysis, including the corresponding tables and charts, are provided in Appendix B, Tables A–C and Figures F–K, available as a supplement to the online version of this article at https://ajph.org.

RESULTS

We constructed a synthetic control for New York's overall firearm mortality, firearm suicide, and firearm homicide rates by utilizing predictive covariates and mortality rates from the period preceding the implementation of the NY SAFE Act. The inclusion of states as synthetic controls was based on their nonzero weights, as summarized in Table 1. Specifically, for the overall firearm mortality, the synthetic controls for New York included California, Hawaii, Maryland, Massachusetts, Nebraska, New Hampshire, Rhode Island, and District of Columbia.

We used RMSPE to evaluate the accuracy of the synthetic controls in approximating New York's firearm mortality rate. Lower RMSPE values signify a better fit.[31,32] As indicated in the last row of Table 1, the synthetic control outperformed the simple average of all states in the donor pool in terms of fit. For instance, in the case of overall firearm mortality, the synthetic control

TABLE 1— Weight Allocation for Synthetic Control Analysis of New York State: 1999–2019

	Weight		
State	Firearm Mortality	Firearm Suicide	Firearm Homicide
Alabama	0.000	0.000	0.000
Alaska	0.000	0.000	0.158
Arizona	0.000	0.000	0.058
Arkansas	0.000	0.000	0.000
California	0.192	0.000	0.000
Connecticut	0.000	0.037	0.000
Delaware	0.000	0.000	0.000
Florida	0.000	0.000	0.000
Georgia	0.000	0.000	0.000
Hawaii	0.305	0.082	0.000
Idaho	0.000	0.000	0.000
Illinois	0.000	0.098	0.000
Kansas	0.000	0.000	0.156
Kentucky	0.000	0.000	0.000
Louisiana	0.000	0.000	0.000
Maine	0.000	0.000	0.000
Maryland	0.031	0.000	0.000
Massachusetts	0.376	0.649	0.017
Minnesota	0.000	0.000	0.123
Mississippi	0.000	0.000	0.000
Missouri	0.000	0.000	0.010
Montana	0.000	0.000	0.000
Nebraska	0.041	0.000	0.000
Nevada	0.000	0.000	0.060
New Hampshire	0.026	0.000	0.000
New Jersey	0.000	0.063	0.000
New Mexico	0.000	0.000	0.000
North Dakota	0.000	0.000	0.000
Ohio	0.000	0.000	0.000
Oklahoma	0.000	0.000	0.000
Oregon	0.000	0.000	0.106
Pennsylvania	0.000	0.071	0.000
Rhode Island	0.012	0.000	0.000
South Carolina	0.000	0.000	0.000
South Dakota	0.000	0.000	0.000
Texas	0.000	0.000	0.000
Utah	0.000	0.000	0.241
Virginia	0.000	0.000	0.064
West Virginia	0.000	0.000	0.000
Wisconsin	0.000	0.000	0.000
Wyoming	0.000	0.000	0.000
Washington, DC	0.017	0.000	0.009
RMSPE synthetic control/all control states	0.159/0.618	0.102/0.424	0.104/0.533

Note. RMSPE = root mean square prediction error. The RMSPE provides a measure of the fit, with lower values indicating a better alignment with New York during the preintervention period.

achieved an RMSPE of 0.159, which is significantly lower than the RMSPE that would have been obtained if a simple average of all control states (i.e., the remaining 49 US states and the District of Columbia) had been used (0.618; Table 1).

Table 2 summarizes the predictive covariates associated with firearm mortality. These variables are presented for both New York and the synthetic control group designed to optimize firearm mortality overall, firearm suicide, and firearm homicide. The similarities in the average balance of these covariates

TABLE 2— Covariate Balance for New York and Synthetic New York State: 1999–2012

	Firearm Mortality		Firearm Suicide		Firearm Homicide	
Covariate	New York	Synthetic New York	New York	Synthetic New York	New York	Synthetic New York
Age, y, %						
< 18 y	20.3	20.4	20.3	19.8	20.3	23.7
≥ 65 y	18.1	18.3	18.1	18.3	18.1	15.6
Female, %	51.1	50.3	51.1	50.8	51.1	49.5
Race/ethnicity, %						
Non-Hispanic White	54.2	47.8	54.2	63.7	54.2	68.7
Non-Hispanic Black	17.7	7.6	17.7	10.1	17.7	6.0
American Indian/Alaska Native	1.0	0.76	1.0	0.5	1.0	3.9
Asian	9.6	17.9	9.6	9.8	9.6	4.9
Pacific Islander	0.1	3.3	0.1	0.9	0.1	0.7
Hispanic	19.7	17.4	19.7	13.9	19.7	13.9
Education level, %						
High school education or lower	87.4	90.4	87.4	91.2	87.4	92.1
Bachelor's degree or higher	38.1	39.3	38.1	40.3	38.1	34.7
Persons in poverty, %	13.9	11.1	13.9	10.7	13.9	10.7
Household income, median, $	75 157.0	86 683.0	75 157.0	85 648.0	75 157.0	74 698.0
Persons without health insurance, %	6.1	5.0	6.1	4.3	6.1	9.9
Unemployment rate, %	3.9	3.3	3.9	3.1	3.9	3.1
Mortality rate,[a] %						
2012	4.8	4.9	2.5	2.6	2.2	2.3
2011	5.0	5.0	2.5	2.4	2.4	2.5
2010	5.1	5.1	2.3	2.5	2.7	2.5
2009	4.8	4.9	2.0	2.0	2.6	2.6
2008	4.9	5.1	2.1	2.2	2.6	2.7
2007	5.1	5.1	2.2	2.2	2.7	2.7
2006	5.2	5.0	2.1	2.0	3.0	2.9
2005	5.3	5.0	2.3	2.1	2.7	2.8
2004	4.9	5.1	2.0	2.0	2.7	2.8
2003	5.3	5.3	2.1	2.2	3.1	3.1
2002	5.1	5.3	2.1	2.1	2.9	2.9
2001	5.5	5.4	2.3	2.3	3.1	3.0
2000	5.7	5.5	2.3	2.3	3.2	3.1
1999	5.3	5.3	2.3	2.4	2.9	3.0

Note. The preintervention period includes 1999–2012, which is the period before the enactment of the NY SAFE Act. Variable balance is assessed by comparing the values in New York (the treatment state) and synthetic New York (its synthetic control). A difference closer to zero indicates better balance between the 2.

[a]Firearm mortality rates are reported per 100 000 population and age-adjusted to the US population in 2000.

serve as further evidence of the close resemblance between the synthetic controls (synthetic New York) and the actual state of New York during the pre–NY SAFE Act period.

We conducted a graphical comparison of the firearm mortality rate over time between New York and synthetic New York. During the preintervention period, before the implementation of the NY SAFE Act, both groups exhibited a closely tracked trajectory, as also supported by the RMSPE of 0.159 and the covariate balance data presented in Table 2. However, starting from 2013, a divergence in rates occurred. While New York's firearm mortality rate continued to decrease through 2019, the rate for synthetic New York increased notably throughout the study period. We compared the rate differences between New York and synthetic New York from 2013 to 2019 and found that the implementation of the NY SAFE Act was associated with a 22.4% reduction in firearm mortality deaths compared with the counterfactual scenario (4.10 vs 5.02; Figure 1; Table 3).

The permutation test results were consistent with the graphical findings, indicating that there was a decrease in New York's overall firearm mortality rate following the implementation of the NY SAFE Act. Furthermore, among the control states with an RMSPE no more than twice that of New York, none exhibited firearm mortality trends that diverged from their synthetic controls to the extent observed in New York (Table 3; Figure A, available as a supplement to the online version of this article at https://ajph.org).

Firearm Suicide

Firearm suicide rates in New York closely tracked those of synthetic New York during the preintervention period. However, a notable divergence between the 2 rates occurred after the implementation of the NY SAFE Act. By summing the differences in rates between New York and synthetic New York from 2013 to 2019, we determined that the NY SAFE Act was linked to 467 fewer deaths than anticipated. However, the permutation test indicated that the observed difference in firearm suicide rates between New York and synthetic New York was not statistically significant and could have occurred by chance (Tables 2 and 3; Appendix A, Figures B and C, available as supplements to the online version of this article at https://ajph.org).

Firearm Homicide

Firearm homicide rates in New York exhibited a close alignment with those of synthetic New York during the preintervention period from 1999 to 2012, as supported by the covariate balance, RMSPE of 0.104, and visual assessments. However, following the implementation of the NY SAFE Act, a divergence in firearm homicide rates occurred, with a continued decrease in New York through

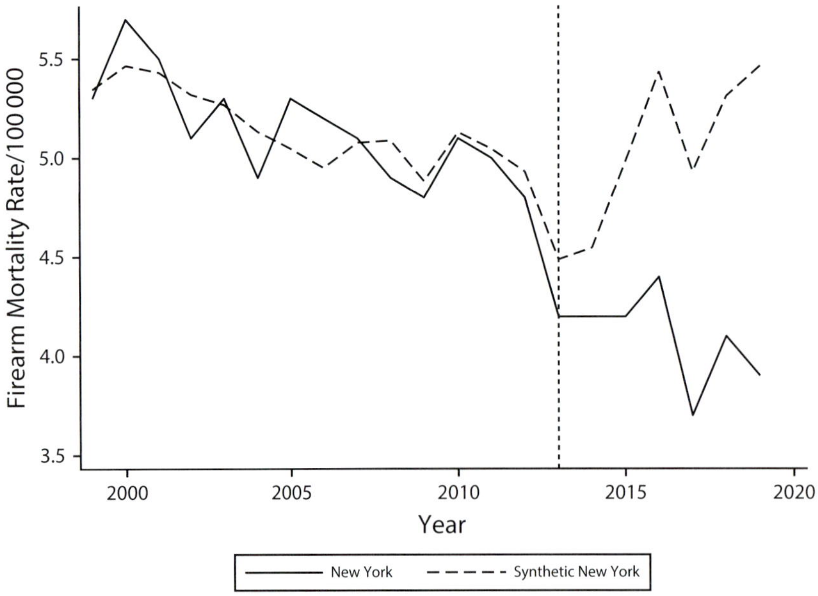

FIGURE 1— Age-Adjusted Firearm Mortality Rate (per 100 000) for New York and Synthetic New York State: 1999–2019

Note. The vertical line indicates the enactment of the New York Secure Ammunition and Firearms Enforcement Act in January 2013.

TABLE 3— Differences in Firearm Mortality Rates for New York State: 1999–2019

	Pre-New York SAFE Act (1999–2012)				Post-New York SAFE Act (2013–2019)				
	New York	Synthetic New York	Relative Change, %	Absolute Difference (95% CI)	New York	Synthetic New York	Relative Change, %	Absolute Difference (95% CI)	Permutation-Based *P*
Firearm mortality	5.14	5.15	0.2	−0.01 (−0.19, 0.17)	4.10	5.02	22.4	−0.92 (−1.29, −0.54)	0.08
Firearm suicide	2.21	2.23	0.9	−0.02 (−0.15, 0.12)	2.12	2.45	15.6	−0.33 (−0.49, 0.17)	0.22
Firearm homicide	2.77	2.78	0.4	−0.01 (−0.21, 0.19)	1.89	3.08	63.0	−1.20 (−1.69, −0.71)	0.026

Note. CI = confidence interval; SAFE = Secure Ammunition and Firearms Enforcement. The *P* value represents the proportion of control units' effects that have posttreatment root mean square prediction error at least as large as the treated unit, while accounting for the quality of pretreatment matches.

2019 and an upward trend in synthetic New York until the end of the study period. The permutation test demonstrated that the difference in postintervention firearm homicide rates between New York and synthetic New York was significant and could not have arisen by chance. From 2013 to 2019, the implementation of the NY SAFE Act is estimated to have prevented a total of 1697 deaths from firearm homicides. This represents a decrease of 63% compared with the counterfactual, with an average rate of 1.89 deaths per 100 000 population as opposed to 3.08 deaths per 100 000 population (Tables 1–3; Appendix A, Figures D and E, available as supplements to the online version of this article at https://ajph.org).

Sensitivity Analysis for Nonfirearm Mortality

To investigate potential substitution effects, we examined the relationship between the NY SAFE Act and nonfirearm mortality overall, nonfirearm suicide, and nonfirearm homicide. The permutation tests conducted indicated that there was no significant association between any of these outcomes and the implementation of the NY SAFE Act (see Appendix B: Tables A–C and Figures F–K, for the detailed results).

DISCUSSION

In this quasi-experimental study, we identified a significant reduction in firearm homicide associated with the implementation of the NY SAFE Act. However, we did not observe an association between the NY SAFE Act and firearm suicide.

The NY SAFE Act, compared with other state firearm laws, incorporates a multitude of comprehensive provisions aimed at reducing gun-related harm.[19] The Act stands out as a multifaceted measure with provisions, including the "1-feature test" for assault weapons, restrictions on large-capacity magazines, mandatory background checks for firearm purchases, and measures to enhance safe storage practices.[19] These provisions collectively address various aspects of firearm safety and access, highlighting the Act's comprehensive approach. While some states have implemented similar provisions individually, the NY SAFE Act goes beyond by encompassing a broader range of measures, making it one of the more comprehensive state laws enacted in recent years.[24] The inclusion of such provisions in the NY SAFE Act likely contributes to the observed reduction in firearm mortality found in this study, reinforcing the importance of comprehensive approaches to gun regulation.

The provision of the NY SAFE Act concerning assault weapons and large-capacity magazines may partially account for the observed decrease in firearm homicide in this study. Section 37 of the Act introduces the "1-feature test," which effectively prohibits semiautomatic weapons with detachable magazines that possess 1 military-related feature.[19] In addition, the Act bans the sale of new large-capacity magazines capable of holding more than 7 rounds of ammunition, with current owners required to transfer such magazines out of state or to firearms dealers.[19] Given that ammunition and large-capacity magazines can contribute to mass shootings, which involve 4 or more victims, regulating the sale and use of these weapons logically has the potential to limit firearm homicides.[16] Previous research examining mass shootings following the expiration of a federal ban on large-capacity magazines and military-style semiautomatic firearms found a significant increase in both the number of incidents and fatalities.[3] A survey of 32 researchers conducted by the *New York Times* on best practices for reducing mass shootings revealed that an assault weapons ban was the most effective measure.[16]

We did not observe a significant association between the implementation of the NY SAFE Act and firearm suicide. Several potential explanations could account for this finding. A notable aspect of the NY SAFE Act is its provision that requires mental health professionals to report individuals they believe may pose a significant risk of harm to themselves or others.[19] This provision has raised concerns regarding its constitutionality and its impact on the principles of the Hippocratic oath and the physician–patient relationship.[20–24] One possible consequence of this provision is that individuals with mental health issues who are contemplating firearm suicide may be deterred from seeking medical care because of the fear of being flagged and reported.[22–24] This fear arises from the potential risk of having their firearm license revoked and their firearms confiscated.[22–24] The presence of this potential deterrent effect may contribute to the absence of a significant protective association between the NY SAFE Act and firearm suicide. These concerns underscore the importance of conducting further examination and fostering discussion regarding the ethical and legal considerations surrounding firearm policy and mental health.

Another potential explanation for the absence of a significant protective association between the NY SAFE Act and firearm suicide could be the presence of a time lag and long-term effects. The impact of the NY SAFE Act on firearm suicides may require a longer period to manifest.[35] Suicide prevention efforts typically involve comprehensive strategies, including improving access to mental health services, fostering community support, and reducing stigma surrounding mental health issues.[35] These multifaceted approaches may have a more delayed and cumulative effect, contrasting the immediate impact of measures targeting homicides.[35] Thus, the complex nature of suicide prevention efforts and the potential time lag involved may contribute to the lack of a detectable association between the NY SAFE Act and firearm suicide.

Further research is warranted to explore the potential effects of the NY SAFE Act on firearm mortality, including specific mechanisms that may explain the observed reduction in firearm homicides but not firearm suicides. Understanding these nuances can inform comprehensive firearm policies.

Limitations and Strengths

This study has some limitations. We used WONDER data, which were exclusively based on death certificate records of US residents.[27] Future studies may consider investigating the association between the NY SAFE Act and firearm injuries, rather than mortality. Second, our use of state-level data precludes individual-level inference—ecologic fallacy. To improve on this limitation, further studies may consider using individual-level data.

This study has several notable strengths that enhance the internal validity and robustness of our findings. First, we employed SCM, an innovative and novel approach to assess the impact of the NY SAFE Act.[25,31,32] Through SCM, we integrated data from multiple control states to construct a synthetic control that closely resembled New York, enabling a rigorous comparison of outcomes before and after implementation of the Act. Furthermore, our study addressed the issue of potential spillover effects from neighboring states by incorporating their data into the donor pool. The synthetic control analysis assigned weights based on similarities to the intervention state, considering factors such as geographic proximity and the potential for contamination.[31,32] Specifically, for overall firearm mortality, states adjacent to New York were assigned a weight of zero and were not included as synthetic controls. In the case of firearm suicide, Connecticut had a weight of 0.037 and New Jersey had a weight of 0.063, indicating their minimal contributions as synthetic controls. Finally, we explored the possibility of substitution effects by examining the association between the NY SAFE Act and nonfirearm suicide and homicide. This comprehensive analysis allowed us to assess whether any reductions in firearm mortality were counterbalanced by increases in non–firearm-related deaths.

Public Health Implications

The implementation of the NY SAFE Act is associated with reduced firearm homicide rates. However, no significant association was observed with firearm suicide rates. As states assume a larger role in enacting firearm policies, our findings provide valuable insights for discussions and considerations on the potential impact of future firearm policies and state-level interventions in reducing firearm-related fatalities in the United States. AJPH

ABOUT THE AUTHORS

Ibraheem M. Karaye, Gaia Knight, and Corinne M. Kyriacou are with the Department of Population Health, Hofstra University, Hempstead, NY.

CORRESPONDENCE

Correspondence should be sent to Ibraheem M. Karaye, MD, DrPH, Department of Population Health, 106 Hofstra Dome, Hofstra University,

Hempstead, NY 11549 (e-mail: ibraheem.m.karaye@hofstra.edu). Reprints can be ordered at https://ajph.org by clicking the "Reprints" link.

PUBLICATION INFORMATION

Full Citation: Karaye IM, Knight G, Kyriacou C. Association between the New York safe act and firearm suicide and homicide: an analysis of synthetic controls, New York State, 1999–2019. *Am J Public Health*. 2023;113(12):1309–1317.

Acceptance Date: July 20, 2023.

DOI: https://doi.org/10.2105/AJPH.2023.307400

CONTRIBUTORS

I. M. Karaye and G. Knight conceptualized and designed the study. I. M. Karaye conducted the analyses. I. M. Karaye, G. Knight, and C. M. Kyriacou drafted the article. C. M. Kyriacou revised the article critically for important intellectual content. All authors provided significant input and approved the final version of the article.

CONFLICTS OF INTEREST

The authors have no relevant financial or nonfinancial interests to disclose.

HUMAN PARTICIPANT PROTECTION

This research was based on publicly accessible and deidentified national data and was deemed exempt from institutional review board review. Because the Centers for Disease Control and Prevention's Wide-ranging Online Data for Epidemiologic Research database provides publicly available and de-identified data, this study was exempted from the institutional review board approval of Hofstra University.

REFERENCES

1. Mangan D. Supreme Court strikes down New York gun law restricting concealed carry in major Second Amendment case. 2022. Available at: https://www.cnbc.com/2022/06/23/supreme-court-strikes-down-new-york-gun-law-restricting-concealed-carry.html. Accessed October 16, 2023.
2. Wilson N. Fact sheet: Weakening requirements to carry a concealed firearm increases violent crime. *American Progress*. 2022. Available at: https://www.americanprogress.org/article/fact-sheet-weakening-requirements-to-carry-a-concealed-firearm-increases-violent-crime. Accessed October 16, 2023.
3. Cook PJ, Donohue JJ. Regulating assault weapons and large-capacity magazines for ammunition. *JAMA*. 2022;328(12):1191–1192. https://doi.org/10.1001/jama.2022.17120
4. Siegel M, Xuan Z, Ross CS, et al. Easiness of legal access to concealed firearm permits and homicide rates in the United States. *Am J Public Health*. 2017;107(12):1923–1929. https://doi.org/10.2105/AJPH.2017.304057
5. Romero MP, Wintemute GJ. The epidemiology of firearm suicide in the United States. *J Urban Health*. 2002;79(1):39–48. https://doi.org/10.1093/jurban/79.1.39
6. American Public Health Association. Gun violence is a public health crisis. 2022. Available at: https://www.apha.org/-/media/files/pdf/factsheets/200221_gun_violence_fact_sheet.ashx. Accessed October 16, 2023.
7. National Center for Health Statistics. Firearm mortality by state. 2022. Available at: https://www.cdc.gov/nchs/pressroom/sosmap/firearm_mortality/firearm.htm. Accessed October 16, 2023.
8. National Center for Health Statistics. Key health indicators. 2022. Available at: https://www.cdc.gov/nchs/pressroom/states/newyork/ny.htm. Accessed October 16, 2023.
9. Every Stat. How does gun violence impact the communities you care about? 2022. Available at: https://everystat.org/#NewYork. Accessed October 16, 2023.
10. Galea S, Abdalla SM. State firearm laws and firearm-related mortality and morbidity. *JAMA*. 2022;328(12):1189–1190. https://doi.org/10.1001/jama.2022.16648
11. Santaella-Tenorio J, Cerdá M, Villaveces A, Galea S. What do we know about the association between firearm legislation and firearm-related injuries [erratum in *Epidemiol Rev*. 2017;39(1):171–172]? *Epidemiol Rev*. 2016;38(1):140–157. https://doi.org/10.1093/epirev/mxv012
12. Lee LK, Fleegler EW, Farrell C, et al. Firearm laws and firearm homicides: a systematic review. *JAMA Intern Med*. 2017;177(1):106–119. https://doi.org/10.1001/jamainternmed.2016.7051
13. Schell TL, Cefalu M, Griffin BA, Smart R, Morral AR. Changes in firearm mortality following the implementation of state laws regulating firearm access and use. *Proc Natl Acad Sci U S A*. 2020;117(26):14906–14910. https://doi.org/10.1073/pnas.1921965117
14. Raifman J, Larson E, Barry CL, et al. State handgun purchase age minimums in the US and adolescent suicide rates: regression discontinuity and difference-in-differences analyses. *BMJ*. 2020;370:m2436. https://doi.org/10.1136/bmj.m2436
15. McCourt AD, Crifasi CK, Stuart EA, et al. Purchaser licensing, point-of-sale background check laws, and firearm homicide and suicide in 4 US states, 1985–2017. *Am J Public Health*. 2020;110(10):1546–1552. https://doi.org/10.2105/AJPH.2020.305822
16. Sanger-Katz M, Bui Q. How to reduce mass shooting deaths? Experts rank gun laws. 2017. Available at: https://www.nytimes.com/interactive/2017/10/05/upshot/how-to-reduce-mass-shooting-deaths-experts-say-these-gun-laws-could-help.html. Accessed October 16, 2023.
17. Crifasi CK, Merrill-Francis M, McCourt A, Vernick JS, Wintemute GJ, Webster DW. Association between firearm laws and homicide in urban counties [erratum in *J Urban Health*. 2018;95(5):773–776]. *J Urban Health*. 2018;95(3):383–390. https://doi.org/10.1007/s11524-018-0273-3
18. Degli Esposti M, Wiebe DJ, Gasparrini A, Humphreys DK. Analysis of "stand your ground" self-defense laws and statewide rates of homicides and firearm homicides [erratum in *JAMA Netw Open*. 2022;5(4):e229270]. *JAMA Netw Open*. 2022;5(2):e220077. https://doi.org/10.1001/jamanetworkopen.2022.0077
19. New York State Senate. Senate Bill S2230. 2013. Available at: https://www.nysenate.gov/legislation/bills/2013/S2230. Accessed October 16, 2023.
20. Gamsin M. The New York SAFE Act: a thoughtful approach to gun control, or a politically expedient response to the public's fear of the mentally ill. *S Cal L Rev Postscript*. 2015;88(2):16–54. Available at: https://southerncalifornialawreview.com/wp-content/uploads/2018/01/88_PS16.pdf. Accessed October 24, 2023.
21. Spitzer RJ. New York State and the New York SAFE Act: a case study in strict gun laws. *Alb L Rev*. 2014;78(2):749–787. Available at: https://www.albanylawreview.org/article/70003-new-york-state-and-the-new-york-safe-act-a-case-study-in-strict-gun-laws. Accessed October 24, 2023.
22. Wiehl T. The presumption of dangerousness: how New York's SAFE Act reflects our irrational fear of mental illness. *Seton Hall Legis J*. 2014;38:35–69. Available at: https://scholarship.shu.edu/shlj/vol38/iss1/3. Accessed October 24, 2023.
23. Eells GT. The implications of New York State's SAFE Act of 2013 on mental health professionals nationally. *J Coll Stud Psychother*. 2013;27(3):177–180. https://doi.org/10.1080/87568225.2013.798207
24. Jacobs JB, Fuhr Z. Was the SAFE Act necessary? In: *The Toughest Gun Control Law in the Nation*. New York, NY: New York University Press; 2019:27–44.
25. Athey S, Imbens GW. The state of applied econometrics: causality and policy evaluation. *J Econ Perspect*. 2017;31(2):3–32. https://doi.org/10.1257/jep.31.2.3
26. Woolf SH, Chapman DA, Lee JH. COVID-19 as the leading cause of death in the United States. *JAMA*. 2021;325(2):123–124. https://doi.org/10.1001/jama.2020.24865
27. Centers for Disease Control and Prevention. About underlying cause of death, 1999–2020. 2022. Available at: https://wonder.cdc.gov/ucd-icd10.html. Accessed October 16, 2023.
28. US Census Bureau. Data. 2022. Available at: https://www.census.gov/data.html. Accessed October 16, 2023.
29. US Bureau of Labor Statistics. Local area unemployment statistics. 2022. Available at: https://www.bls.gov/web/laus/laumstrk.htm. Accessed October 16, 2023.
30. Esposti MD, Wiebe D, Kaufman E, Bonander C. Synthetic control methodology for examining firearm policy. *Curr Epidemiol Rep*. 2022;9(3):109–125. https://doi.org/10.1007/s40471-022-00294-9
31. Abadie A, Diamond A, Hainmueller J. Synthetic control methods for comparative case studies: estimating the effect of California's tobacco control program. *J Am Stat Assoc*. 2010;105(490):493–505. https://doi.org/10.1198/jasa.2009.ap08746
32. Abadie A, Diamond A, Hainmueller J. Comparative politics and the synthetic control method. *Am J Pol Sci*. 2015;59(2):495–510. https://doi.org/10.1111/ajps.12116
33. Chrisinger BW. Philadelphia's excise tax on sugar-sweetened and artificially sweetened beverages and supplemental nutrition assistance program benefit redemption. *Am J Public Health*. 2021;111(11):1986–1996. https://doi.org/10.2105/AJPH.2021.306464
34. Galiani S, Quistorff B. The synth_runner package: utilities to automate synthetic control estimation using synth. *Stata J*. 2017;17(4):834–849. https://doi.org/10.1177/1536867X1801700404
35. Mann JJ, Michel CA. Prevention of firearm suicide in the United States: what works and what is possible. *Am J Psychiatry*. 2016;173(10):969–979. https://doi.org/10.1176/appi.ajp.2016.16010069

Child Mental Health Status in Flint, Michigan: A Worsening Health Inequity, 2018–2022

Jacqueline Dannis, MA, Sarah Jenuwine, BS, Nicole Jones, PhD, MS, Jenny LaChance, MS, CCRC, and Mona Hanna-Attisha, MD, MPH

Objectives. To determine the burden of mental health disorders among children enrolled in Michigan's Flint Registry in the context of a local public health crisis and a nationally declared pediatric mental health crisis.

Methods. This survey-based study included 1203 children aged 3 to 17 years whose caregivers enrolled them in the Flint Registry between December 2018 and March 2020 and who completed a follow-up survey between October 2020 and March 2022. The baseline and follow-up surveys included caregiver reports of childhood anxiety and depression and overall mental health wellness.

Results. At enrollment, Flint Registry caregivers reported significantly higher rates of anxiety and depression among their children than caregivers reported nationally (12.9% vs 9.4% and 8.2% vs 4.4%; $P < .001$). Flint Registry caregivers also reported declines in their children's overall mental health wellness at follow-up, $t(1472) = -4.17$; $P < .001$.

Conclusions. Our findings reveal a disparate burden of pediatric mental health disorders and exemplify the health inequities vulnerable populations face.

Public Health Implications. More proactive and preventive steps should be taken to lessen this burden, especially in chronically disadvantaged communities that experience public health crises. (*Am J Public Health*. 2023;113(12):1318–1321. https://doi.org/10.2105/AJPH.2023.307406)

AJPH December 2023, Vol 113, No. 12

In 2021, the US Centers for Disease Control and Prevention (CDC), the American Academy of Pediatrics, and the Office of the Surgeon General acknowledged a national pediatric mental health emergency. Between 2010 and 2020, rates of childhood anxiety and depression increased steadily.[1] In 2019, 1 in 3 high school students reported persistent feelings of sadness or hopelessness; by 2021, that figure reached 42%.[2,3] Longitudinal studies have shown that childhood anxiety or depression can stem from genetic factors and experiences of trauma, maltreatment, or other early adversities.[4]

From April 2014 through October 2015, the Flint, Michigan, community was exposed to unsafe drinking water with the risk of elevated blood lead levels. Lead exposure has mental and behavioral health consequences, as does exposure to the trauma of an environmental disaster.[5–7] Furthermore, pediatric mental health worsened during the COVID-19 pandemic as a result of social isolation, family economic hardship, family loss or illness, and reduced health care access.[8]

Established before the COVID-19 pandemic, the CDC-supported Flint Registry has engaged in voluntary survey-based population-level surveillance and support for individuals exposed to the Flint water crisis. Enrollment for the Flint Registry began in December 2018, and individuals were recruited through an extensive community-based outreach and marketing campaign.

Recognizing the need to better understand the mental health implications of lead exposure and trauma in the context of a global pandemic, we sought to answer the following question: Considering the national trends in pediatric mental health, what is the mental health status of Flint Registry children? Also, we sought to determine how their mental health status has changed over time.

METHODS

This study included 1203 children aged 3 to 17 years whose caregivers completed a baseline enrollment Flint Registry survey between December 2018 and March 2020 and a follow-up survey between October 2020 and March 2022. The mean (±SD) interval between the completion of the baseline and follow-up surveys was 16 months (±5 months). The children were Flint residents during the water crisis (April 25, 2014, to October 15, 2015), and 88% of caregivers reported that their child was exposed to unfiltered City of Flint tap water during the crisis. Michigan Department of Health and Human Services records were used to verify the identities of the child participants.

Extracted survey data included questions from or adapted from the National Survey of Children's Health: Has a doctor, other health care provider, or educator (such as a teacher or school nurse) ever told you that your child has anxiety problems? Has a doctor, other health care provider, or educator (such as a teacher or school nurse) ever told you that your child has depression? During the past 12 months, has your child received any treatment or counseling from a mental health professional? We compared rates of childhood anxiety and depression among Flint children with CDC data gathered via the same National Survey of Children's Health questions.[9]

In addition, data on overall child mental health were included: In general, would you say your child's mental health is excellent, very good, good, fair, or poor? Information on age, biological sex, free and reduced-cost meal services, and race was also collected.

The survey data were collected via REDCap electronic data capture tools hosted at Michigan State University.[10] SPSS 27 (SPSS Inc, Chicago, IL) was used to analyze the data with 1-sample χ^2, paired sample proportions, and paired *t* tests.

Data were missing for less than 3% of the demographic variables (Table 1). Missing data for the outcome variables anxiety, depression, and parents' reports of overall mental health wellness and treatment ranged from 5% to 8%, and thus our analysis included SPSS multiple imputation for these variables; pooled values are reported.

RESULTS

The mean (±SD) age of the 1203 children at enrollment was 9.0 (±3.7) years. About half of the children (46.6%) were female, and 79.7% were eligible for free or reduced-cost school meals. Most caregivers reported that their child identified as Black or African American only (61.2%); 22.8% reported White only, 1% reported Native American or Alaska Native only, and 12.6% reported more than 1 race.

At enrollment, Flint Registry caregivers reported significantly higher rates of anxiety and depression among their children than in the general population (as reported in 2019 by the CDC[9]), $\chi^2(1, n = 1203) = 17.04$; $P < .001$ and $\chi^2(1, n = 1203) = 41.76$; $P < .001$, respectively. At baseline, 12.9% of the study participants reported anxiety and 8.2% reported depression (as compared with the national rates of 9.4% and 4.4%, respectively[9]).

The percentages of children with anxiety and depression did not change significantly at follow-up. However, caregivers reported a decline in the rating of their child's overall mental health, $t(1472) = -4.17$; $P < .001$. A total of 16.9% of caregivers reported their child's mental health as fair or poor at follow-up, as compared with 14.5% at baseline.

At follow-up, most (54.3%) caregivers reported that children with anxiety or depression had received treatment or counseling from a mental health professional in the preceding 12 months; 13.5% reported that their child had not received treatment or counseling from a mental health professional in the past 12 months but believed that the child needed to see a mental health professional, and 32.2% reported that their child did not need to see a mental health professional. These figures are not significantly different from reported mental health care access rates at baseline (54.7%, 12.8%, and 32.5%, respectively).

DISCUSSION

In this large cohort of children enrolled in the Flint Registry, the findings reveal an outsized burden of pediatric mental health disorders. National trends have prompted declarations of emergency, and our local data reflect even greater alarm and exemplify the health inequities that certain populations face.

Our data may reflect the pathogenesis of exposure to lead and trauma as well as historic and systemic adversity. This study mirrors research on behavioral and mental health outcomes among children in communities affected by manmade environmental disasters.[5–7]

The results of our study do not reveal increases in childhood anxiety and depression after the onset of the

TABLE 1— Flint Registry Children at Enrollment (December 2018–March 2020) Versus National Sample (2019) and at Follow-Up Survey (October 2020–March 2022): Flint, MI

Study Participant Demographics	Mean ±SD, No. (%), or Percentage Point Difference	Significance
Age, y	9 ± 3.7	
Biological sex		
Female	561 (46.6)	
Male	638 (53.0)	
Missing	4 (0.3)	
Free or reduced-cost meals		
No	213 (17.7)	
Yes	959 (79.7)	
Missing	31 (2.6)	
Race		
Black only	736 (61.2)	
White only	274 (22.8)	
Other minority only	12 (1.0)	
More than 1	151 (12.6)	
Missing	30 (2.5)	
Flint vs national sample		
Anxiety	3.5	$\chi^2(1, n = 1203) = 17.04$; $P < .001$
Depression	3.8	$\chi^2(1, n = 1203) = 41.76$; $P < .001$
Change at follow-up		
% with anxiety[a]	−0.8	95% CI = −0.01, 0.03; $P = .446$
% with depression[a]	−0.2	95% CI = −0.01, 0.02; $P = .762$
% receiving treatment[a]	−0.4	95% CI = −0.06, 0.07; $P = .922$
% with poor or fair mental health	2.4	$t(1472) = -4.17$; $P < .001$

Note. CI = confidence interval. Percentages may not sum to 100 owing to rounding. The sample size was 1203.
Source. National sample data are from Bitsko et al.[9]
[a]Tested with paired sample proportion tests.

pandemic, but they do show a worsening of parent-reported overall mental health wellness. This may reflect the impact of the pandemic on the services needed to diagnose new cases of anxiety and depression.

Crisis mitigation efforts in Flint included universal early intervention, mindfulness programming, high-quality child care, Medicaid expansion, parenting support, literacy programming, trauma-informed care, and nutrition services. The effects of these efforts on our findings are unknown. More research is needed.

The limitations of this study rest largely on the registry as a voluntary surveillance tool. In addition, we used a cross-sectional design, and therefore causal inferences cannot be made. The strengths of the study are that the sample size was large and that participants' demographic characteristics mirrored those of the Flint population.

PUBLIC HEALTH IMPLICATIONS

This study of a marginalized population of children is consistent with and supports national efforts to amplify pediatric mental health concerns and encourage early identification. New US Preventive Services Task Force recommendations for anxiety screening of all children beginning at 8 years of age[11] are promising; however, more proactive and preventative steps should be taken to lessen this burden, especially in communities such as Flint that have experienced long-standing systemic inequities atop manmade environmental disasters.[6] Our data also support the expansion of early mental health screening and treatment of mental health disorders, particularly in partnership with local schools, which has been shown to increase receipt of care.[12] AJPH

ABOUT THE AUTHORS

The authors are with the Michigan State University–Hurley Children's Hospital Pediatric Public Health Initiative, Charles Stewart Mott Department of Public Health, Michigan State University College of Human Medicine, Flint.

CORRESPONDENCE

Correspondence should be sent to Jacqueline Dannis, MA, Pediatric Public Health Initiative, Michigan State University College of Human Medicine, 200 East 1st St, Flint, MI 48502 (e-mail: dannis@msu.edu). Reprints can be ordered at http://www.ajph.org by clicking the "Reprints" link.

PUBLICATION INFORMATION

Full Citation: Dannis J, Jenuwine S, Jones N, LaChance J, Hanna-Attisha M. Child mental health status in Flint, Michigan: a worsening health inequity, 2018–2022. *Am J Public Health*. 2023;113(12): 1318–1321.

Acceptance Date: July 27, 2023.

DOI: https://doi.org/10.2105/AJPH.2023.307406

CONTRIBUTORS

J. Dannis originated and supervised the study, performed the data analysis, and led the writing. S. Jenuwine assisted with the study, data analysis, and writing. N. Jones, J. LaChance, and M. Hanna-Attisha designed the Flint Registry. All of the authors interpreted the data and critically revised the article.

ACKNOWLEDGMENTS

This secondary analysis of data was not supported by external funding. Data collected in the Flint Registry project were used in our study. The Flint Registry was supported by grant funding from the Centers for Disease Control and Prevention (CDC; award NUE2EH001370) for an award totaling $20,360,339, with 0% financed with nongovernmental sources; the Genesee County (Michigan) Health Department through the Healthy Start project (grant U62MC31100) from the Health Resources and Services Administration (HRSA) for an award totaling $3,255,399, with 0% financed with nongovernmental sources; and the State of Michigan Department of Education.

This work was presented at the American Public Health Association 2022 Annual Meeting and Expo.

We thank Katlin Harwood-Schelb and Katherine Negele for their assistance with the preparation of the article.

Note. The contents are those of the authors and do not necessarily represent the official views of, or an endorsement by, the CDC, the Genesee County Health Department, HRSA, the US government, or the State of Michigan Department of Education.

CONFLICTS OF INTEREST

Mona Hanna-Attisha is an author (*What The Eyes Don't See*) and speaker and has provided testimony during congressional hearings as a child health expert. The other authors declare no conflicts of interest.

HUMAN PARTICIPANT PROTECTION

The Michigan State University institutional review board approved this secondary analysis of Flint Registry data.

REFERENCES

1. American Academy of Pediatrics. AAP-AACAP-CHA declaration of a national emergency in child and adolescent mental health. Available at: https://www.aap.org/en/advocacy/child-and-adolescent-healthy-mental-development/aap-aacap-cha-declaration-of-a-national-emergency-in-child-and-adolescent-mental-health. Accessed June 20, 2023.
2. Centers for Disease Control and Prevention. Youth Risk Behavior Survey data summary and trends report: 2009–2019. Available at: https://www.cdc.gov/healthyyouth/data/yrbs/pdf/YRBSDataSummaryTrendsReport2019-508.pdf. Accessed June 20, 2023.
3. Centers for Disease Control and Prevention. Youth Risk Behavior Survey data summary and trends report: 2011–2021. Available at: https://www.cdc.gov/healthyyouth/data/yrbs/pdf/YRBS_Data-Summary-Trends_Report2023_508.pdf. Accessed June 20, 2023.
4. Franić S, Middeldorp CM, Dolan CV, Ligthart L, Boomsma DI. Childhood and adolescent anxiety and depression: beyond heritability. *J Am Acad Child Adolesc Psychiatry*. 2010;49(8):820–829. https://doi.org/10.1016/j.jaac.2010.05.013
5. Jones N, Dannis J, O'Connell L, LaChance J, LeWinn K, Hanna-Attisha M. Parent report of child behaviour: findings from the Flint Registry cohort. *Paediatr Perinat Epidemiol*. 2022;36(5): 750–758. https://doi.org/10.1111/ppe.12888
6. Chung S, Kim E. Physical and mental health of disaster victims: a comparative study on typhoon and oil spill disasters. *J Prev Med Public Health*. 2010;43(5):387–395. https://doi.org/10.3961/jpmph.2010.43.5.387
7. Fortenberry GZ, Reynolds P, Burrer SL, et al. Assessment of behavioral health concerns in the community affected by the Flint water crisis—Michigan (USA) 2016. *Prehosp Disaster Med*. 2018;33(3):256–265. https://doi.org/10.1017/S1049023X18000250
8. Jones SE, Ethier KA, Hertz M, et al. Mental health, suicidality, and connectedness among high school students during the COVID-19 pandemic—Adolescent Behaviors and Experiences Survey, United States, January–June 2021. *MMWR Suppl*. 2022;71(3):16–21. https://doi.org/10.15585/mmwr.su7103a3
9. Bitsko RH, Claussen AH, Lichstein J, et al. Mental health surveillance among children—United States, 2013–2019. *MMWR Suppl*. 2022;71(2): 1–42. https://doi.org/10.15585/mmwr.su7102a1
10. Harris PA, Taylor R, Thielke R, Payne J, Gonzalez N, Conde JG. Research electronic data capture (REDCap)—a metadata-driven methodology and workflow process for providing translational research informatics support. *J Biomed Inform*. 2009;42(2):377–381. https://doi.org/10.1016/j.jbi.2008.08.010
11. US Preventive Services Task Force. Screening for anxiety in children and adolescents: US Preventive Services Task Force recommendation statement. *JAMA*. 2022;328(14):1438–1444. https://doi.org/10.1001/jama.2022.16936
12. Dittus PJ, De Rosa CJ, Jeffries RA, et al. The Project Connect health systems intervention: linking sexually experienced youth to sexual and reproductive health care. *J Adolesc Health*. 2014;55(4):528–534. https://doi.org/10.1016/j.jadohealth.2014.04.005

Employee Cardiometabolic Risk Following a Cluster-Randomized Workplace Intervention From the Work, Family and Health Network, 2009–2013

Lisa F. Berkman, PhD, Erin L. Kelly, PhD, Leslie B. Hammer, PhD, Frank Mierzwa, PMP, Todd Bodner, PhD, Tay McNamara, PhD, Hayami K. Koga, MD, PhD, Soomi Lee, PhD, Miguel Marino, PhD, Laura C. Klein, PhD, Thomas W. McDade, PhD, Ginger Hanson, PhD, Phyllis Moen, PhD, and Orfeu M. Buxton, PhD

AJPH December 2023, Vol 113, No. 12

Objectives. To examine whether workplace interventions to increase workplace flexibility and supervisor support and decrease work–family conflict can reduce cardiometabolic risk.

Methods. We randomly assigned employees from information technology (n = 555) and long-term care (n = 973) industries in the United States to the Work, Family and Health Network intervention or usual practice (we collected the data 2009–2013). We calculated a validated cardiometabolic risk score (CRS) based on resting blood pressure, HbA_{1c} (glycated hemoglobin), HDL (high-density lipoprotein) and total cholesterol, height and weight (body mass index), and tobacco consumption. We compared changes in baseline CRS to 12-month follow-up.

Results. There was no significant main effect on CRS associated with the intervention in either industry. However, significant interaction effects revealed that the intervention improved CRS at the 12-month follow-up among intervention participants in both industries with a higher baseline CRS. Age also moderated intervention effects: older employees had significantly larger reductions in CRS at 12 months than did younger employees.

Conclusions. The intervention benefited employee health by reducing CRS equivalent to 5 to 10 years of age-related changes for those with a higher baseline CRS and for older employees.

Trial Registration. ClinicalTrials.gov Identifier: NCT02050204. (*Am J Public Health*. 2023;113(12): 1322–1331. https://doi.org/10.2105/AJPH.2023.307413)

Work is a key social determinant of health and well-being and provides many opportunities and resources as well as exposures to health risks. It is central in shaping inequalities in health. One of the key organizational conditions shaping workplace risk or protection is the ability to go to work without creating undue hardship and strain on family responsibilities and obligations, thus determining work–family conflict.[1] Work–family conflict is of growing concern in the United States, as the majority of women with younger children work outside the home and more workers need to care for older adults, including parents, partners, close friends, and family.[2,3] Dual wage–earning families are common, potentially increasing work demands for the entire family and reducing opportunities for home care. As a result, men and women increasingly experience major work and family responsibilities.

About 70% of US workers report some interference between work and nonwork.[4] Such interference is reported to degrade employee health, but few experimental approaches have been used and even fewer had strong disease biomarkers. Furthermore, recent workplace wellness program studies using strong randomized designs reported limited positive results,[5–7] including some improvements in health behaviors and intentions to change behaviors but no differences in clinical or self-reported health outcomes[5–7]or medical or pharmaceutical spending or utilization.[7] In this light, it is important to consider workplace redesign practices that directly influence stressful workplace conditions.[8] This perspective is aligned with a social determinants of health approach in which the work itself—how it is organized and structured—shapes risks for health and well-being.

Rather than viewing the workplace as a venue for delivering health care or wellness benefits implicitly or explicitly asking workers to manage their stress as individuals, we see work and the structure of the workplace as a potential determinant of health.[9] Our framework focuses on reducing toxic environments, not on asking workers to adapt to risky working conditions. By using strong randomized experimental designs, such as what we used in this study, we can better assess causal impacts of changing workplace conditions on health, in this case cardiometabolic disease risk.

Previous systematic reviews[10–13] of observational studies have linked work stress to mortality and cardiovascular morbidity, and several studies from the Work, Family and Health Network (WFHN) have linked work–family conflict to health and cardiovascular risks.[14,15] A pilot supervisor support intervention was associated with decreases in blood pressure.[15] The WFHN intervention positively affected objectively measured sleep, recently recognized by the American Heart Association as important for heart health.[16] In systematic reviews and meta-analyses,[11,17] risks were found to be about 1.2 and somewhat higher (1.3) when issues of reverse causality were addressed. Selection into more stressful jobs related to preexisting poor health, low educational attainment, or other sources of disadvantage may still affect results.[15,18] Both confounding by other conditions and selection into stressful jobs reduces confidence in observational studies; experimental designs are needed for strong causal inference.

Biological mechanisms underlying the link between work stress and cardiovascular disease include coagulation, inflammation, and cardiovascular reactivity[13] as well as atherosclerosis and general metabolic syndromes,[19] but the strongest links between job strain and cardiovascular risk rest largely on prospective epidemiologic studies. However, as noted by Kivimäki and Kawachi, "The strongest evidence for causation derives from experimental manipulation of the exposure (work stress) to see whether it can affect outcomes of interest. Experimental evidence of this sort remains extremely sparse in the area of work stress."[19(p2)]

We provide experimental evidence that a workplace intervention designed to increase employee control over work time, train supervisors to support personal and family life, and reduce low-value work that leads to workers feeling overloaded can improve employees' cardiovascular health.

The WFHN designed a group-randomized experiment to intervene in work conditions to improve cardiovascular health, mental health, sleep, and workplace productivity.[20] We report on the primary aim related to cardiovascular risk in 2 different industries: the long term care industry and an information technology (IT) industry. These 2 industries with their different wages and occupations provide an opportunity to test the intervention in distinct contexts.

The workplace intervention was designed to increase family-supportive supervisor behaviors and employee control over work time to decrease work–family conflict and improve health.[21,22] We hypothesized that the intervention would decrease employees' risk of developing cardiovascular disease, which was assessed by a validated cardiometabolic risk score (CRS).[23]

We tested a secondary hypothesis: that the effect of the intervention on cardiometabolic risk would be moderated by baseline cardiometabolic risk and age.[24] We reasoned that intervention effects would be more apparent for vulnerable employees with higher baseline cardiometabolic risk or who were older. Younger employees with lower baseline cardiometabolic risk would not benefit as much in terms of risk reduction although they may have benefited in terms of other outcomes, such as psychological distress.[25]

METHODS

The group-randomized experimental study design has been described previously[14,22,26] and registered, with our primary cardiovascular outcome the change in the modified Framingham risk score from baseline to 12 months follow-up (we collected data 2009–2013). We recruited participants from 2 companies with multiple work sites (long-term care facilities) or multiple work units (IT) in the United States. Employees were eligible to participate if they were at least 18 years old. Each participant provided written informed consent and completed a baseline preintervention survey with biomarker collection. Follow-up assessments included in-person interviews and biomarker collection. Our analytic sample for cardiovascular risk consisted of individuals with both baseline and 12-month postintervention follow-up data, of whom there were 973 in long-term care and 555 in IT, as specified in our registration with

ClinicalTrials.gov. Figure 1 is the CONSORT (consolidated standards of reporting trials) diagram, which shows each study step with its associated sample size. The unit of randomization was the worksite or work unit, not the individual.

We evaluated measurements at 2 time points: baseline (preintervention) and our major endpoint (the 12-month postintervention follow-up). Recruitment spanned September 2009 to July 2011. One company consisted largely of female, low-wage direct care workers and the other company consisted of male and female high- and moderate-salaried technical workers. We randomly assigned work units to either intervention or usual practice using an adaptive randomization technique[27] modified for each industry.[26] For long-term care, facilities or nursing homes (n = 30) were the units of randomization. For the IT industry, work units analogous to departments were the units of randomization (n = 56). All regular employees in IT groups were eligible to participate. In long-term care, direct care workers (e.g., registered nurses, certified nursing assistants) who worked for 22.5 hours or more per week on at least some day shifts were eligible to participate. We calculated power for estimated intervention effects on the modified Framingham score based on pilot work,[28] conservatively concluding that we had sufficient power to detect effects with 15 groups per condition and a minimum sample size of 20 employees per group.

Recruitment materials emphasized describing connections between employees' working conditions and health. Trained study site managers introduced the study to employees and coordinated project implementation. To minimize bias, using separate and blinded field interviewers, we obtained informed consent and collected data from employees in intervention and usual practice groups at baseline and follow-up. We collected baseline data approximately 1 month before intervention. We collected self-reported measures with a 60-minute computer-assisted personal interview at each time point. We describe biomarkers, including blood pressure measures, dried blood spots for HbA_{1c} and cholesterol, and weight and height measures for body mass index in the "Study Outcomes" section. Employees received up to $60 for completing data collection.

Study Oversight

A data safety and monitoring board reviewed the trial. Work, Family and Health steering committee members

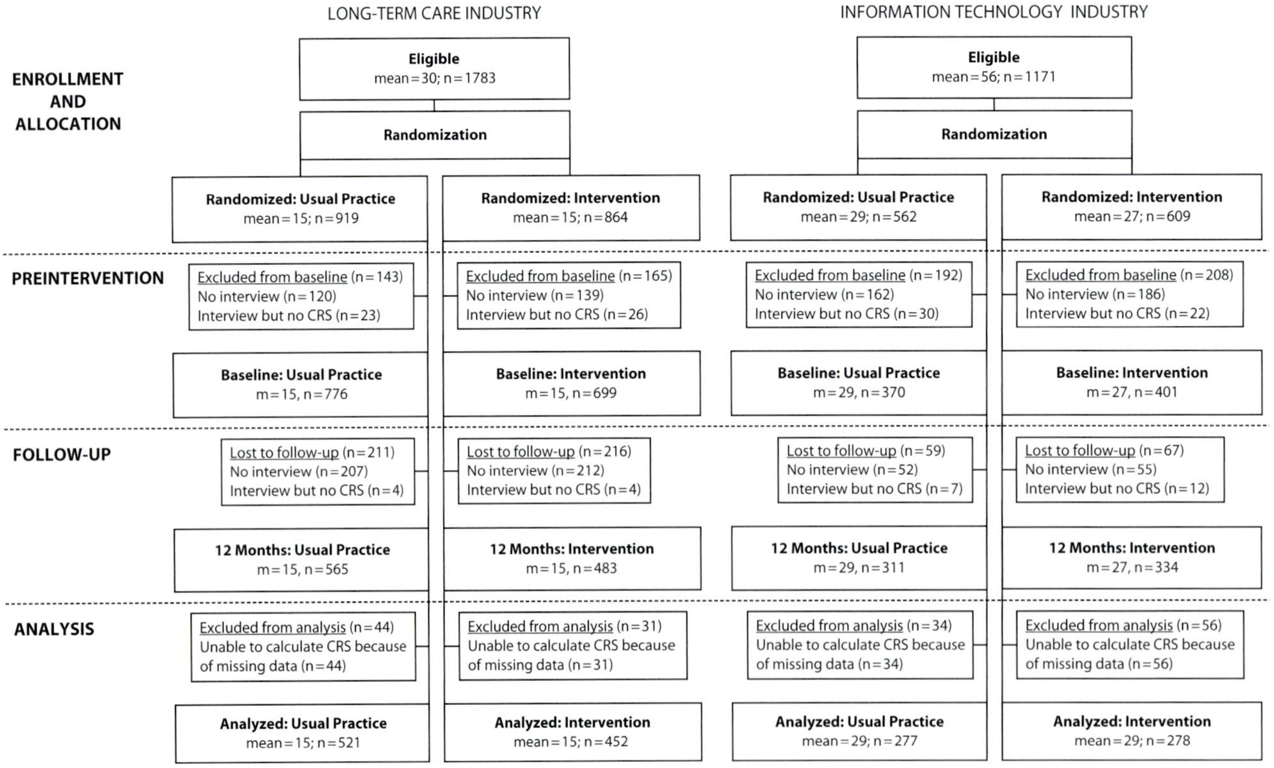

FIGURE 1— CONSORT Diagram: United States, 2009–2013

Note. CRS = cardiometabolic risk score; mean = mean cluster size.

who oversaw the trial can attest that the study was performed in accordance with protocols and the statistical analysis plan and vouch for accuracy and completeness of reported analyses.

Study Intervention

The intervention consisted of supervisor training focused on increasing supportive work–family behaviors and work redesign activities aimed to modify practices and interactions in workplaces between employees and their direct supervisors. The intervention was a structural and social change process designed specifically to increase employees' control over work time and supervisors' awareness and support of work–family balance; the intervention integrated pilot interventions that independently improved employee health.[29,30] Frontline managers participated in online and in-person training on strategies to demonstrate support for employees' personal and family lives while supporting employees' job performance. Employees and managers attended participatory training sessions where teams identified new work practices to increase employees' control over work time and to help reduce low-value tasks. Intervention activities unfolded over 12 weeks. We invited nonsupervisory employees to between 5 hours (in long-term care) and 7.5 hours (in IT) of training, and we invited managers to 4 additional hours of training.[21,22] Detailed training and support materials are available online (https://workfamilyhealthnetwork.org).

Study Outcomes

The primary outcome was CRS, a sex-stratified and validated score in the Framingham Offspring cohort to predict subsequent 10-year cardiovascular event risk.[23] We created the score using sex-specific algorithms based on 6 biomarkers:

1. systolic blood pressure (mm Hg),
2. body mass index (kg/m^2),
3. glycated hemoglobin (HbA_{1c}, %),
4. tobacco consumption (smoker vs nonsmoker),
5. HDL (high-density lipoprotein) cholesterol (mg/dl), and
6. total cholesterol (mg/dl).

We calculated scores for respondents who had both baseline and 12-month assessments. Higher scores indicate higher estimated risk (%) of developing cardiovascular disease 10 years later. We conducted study-specific equivalency analyses on dried blood spot biomarkers and included control values in shipments to the biomarker laboratory for this specific purpose. We used these serum equivalencies for dried blood spot measures.[31]

Statistical Analysis

Summaries of continuous variables are presented as means ±SDs for normally distributed data and as frequencies (percentages) for categorical variables. We compared baseline covariates between study groups by using the χ^2 test for categorical variables and the Student *t* test for continuous variables.[26]

We performed analyses on complete cases separately for each of the 2 industries, resulting in 4 models (an overall intervention effect model for each industry and a moderation analysis by baseline CRS for each industry). For all 4 models, we performed analyses at the participant level, using linear mixed effects models to estimate the mean between-group difference in 10-year cardiovascular risk from baseline to 12 months. All models included random effects for participants to account for temporal correlation and random effects for workgroups to account for clustering of participants in workgroups.

To assess the overall impact of the intervention on 10-year cardiovascular risk, we followed a difference-in-difference approach that included an indicator for time (with baseline set as the reference), an indicator for intervention group (with usual practice serving as the reference), and the interaction between time and intervention. The effect of the intervention was represented by a 2-way interaction model parameter that represented the difference in relative average difference in CRS between intervention individuals relative to usual practice individuals across time. In addition to these terms, for long-term care, we included a control for the number of employees in a cluster. For the IT cohort, we also included the number of employees in a cluster and categorical indicators of unit function (core or support), whether that unit's baseline data were collected before or after a major organizational change (a merger) was announced, and a categorical indicator of whether the unit was reorganized during the study period.

We intended these control variables to address potential structural differences between treatment and control groups that randomization might not have fully addressed. Our analysis suggests that other potential differences, such as race and gender, between treatment and control groups were slight, and replications of analyses with controls adjusting for any differences in those characteristics were consistent with the main analysis.

To test the a priori hypothesis that the effect of the intervention on 10-year cardiovascular risk would be moderated by baseline CRS risk, we adapted linear mixed models to include a 3-way interaction for the moderating variable of interest (baseline CRS). The 3-way interaction parameter represented the moderating effect of baseline CRS risk on the difference in relative average difference in outcomes between intervention individuals relative to usual practice individuals across time after controlling for potential confounders. We assessed evidence of any differential intervention effects on the primary outcome with the use of a likelihood ratio test for the 3-way interaction term.

As a sensitivity analysis, we also conducted intent-to-treat with last observation carried forward for those with missing data at the 12-month follow-up. All statistical tests were 2-sided, and statistical significance was defined at $P < .05$. We performed statistical analyses in SAS version 9.3 (SAS Institute, Cary, NC).

RESULTS

Table 1 shows the characteristics of participants by industry and intervention conditions. Overall, treatment and control groups were well balanced in terms of sociodemographic and health characteristics for both industries. In long-term care, control group respondents were slightly older, and a larger proportion were Hispanic and foreign born compared with respondents in the intervention group. In the IT cohort, a larger proportion of control group respondents were Asian/Pacific Islander (difference = 19) and foreign-born; the number of participants in these categories was small and did not influence results. Attrition rate did not differ by treatment group in either industry (Figure 1). Participants lost to follow-up were similar in treatment and control groups in the long-term care sample. In IT, participants lost to follow-up were slightly younger (no difference by treatment group) and slightly less likely to be non-Hispanic White and native-born (data available on request).

We estimated the amount of the intervention received by employee intervention session attendance. In IT, intervention sessions were attended by 75% of the analytic sample; 9% of employees (n = 25) attended fewer than half of the sessions, and 4% (n = 10) attended no sessions. In long-term care, intervention sessions were attended by 67% of the analytic sample; 29% of employees (n = 122) attended fewer than half of the sessions, and 9% (n = 38) attended no sessions.

Intervention Effects on Cardiometabolic Risk Score

Table 2 presents results from the evaluation of the overall intervention effects on CRS by industry. We present CRS by intervention and usual practice for each industry at baseline and 12 months with 95% confidence intervals (CIs). Although CRS in both usual practice groups at 12 months were slightly higher than at baseline, and CRS in intervention groups were slightly lower, the CIs overlap. We observed no statistically significant intervention main effect in either industry (reduction in CRS in the long-term care industry cohort: B = −0.27; 95% CI = −0.63, 0.08; in the IT cohort: B = −0.21; 95% CI = −0.62, 0.20).

Effects by Baseline Cardiometabolic Risk Score

In prespecified subgroup analyses, we compared intervention impacts on workers who had higher baseline CRS. Baseline CRS moderated intervention effects (Table 2). For both industries, intervention employees who had higher CRS at baseline exhibited significant decreases in CRS at 12-month follow-up (Figure 2). Specifically, the intervention decreased CRS for long-term care workers (B = −0.08; 95% CI = −0.13, −0.04) and for IT workers (B = −0.07; 95% CI = −0.12, −0.01) whose baseline CRS was higher. To put the effect magnitude into perspective, we express these differences relative to age-related differences in risk. In supplementary analyses, magnitudes of effects for the average worker (−0.31 for long-term care and −0.18 for IT) were comparable with age-related increases in CRS equivalent to 5.5 years in the IT cohort and 10.3 years in the long-term care cohort.

Intervention Effects by Age

In supplementary analyses, we found that these effects were more apparent in older employees. Figure A (available as a supplement to the online version of this article at http://www.ajph.org) shows that older employees (≥ 45 years) who had higher CRS at baseline were more likely to decrease CRS at 12 months than were younger employees (< 45 years) who also had higher CRS at baseline. Note that older employees had higher CRS at baseline on average than younger employees.

In the intention-to-treat analyses shown in Table A (available as a supplement to the online version of this article at http://www.ajph.org), results were qualitatively similar to those of the complete case analyses. In particular, main effect terms remained nonsignificant, and the CRS moderating effects were similar in magnitude and statistical significance (IT: $P = .01$; long-term care: $P < .001$).

TABLE 1— Selected Characteristics of Study Participants by Industry: United States, 2009–2013

	Long-Term Care			IT		
	Intervention (n = 452), Mean ±SD or No. (%)	Control (n = 521), Mean ±SD or No. (%)	Δ	Intervention (n = 278), Mean ±SD or No. (%)	Control (n = 277), Mean ±SD or No. (%)	Δ
Baseline sociodemographics						
Age, y	37.7 ± 12.4	39.6 ± 12.1	*	46.6 ± 8.9	46.1 ± 8.6	
Male sex	34 (7.5)	47 (9.0)		160 (57.6)	173 (62.5)	
Married/partnered	277 (61.3)	341 (65.5)		224 (80.6)	222 (80.1)	
Caregiver	140 (31.0)	149 (28.6)		66 (23.7)	65 (23.5)	
Race/ethnicity						
White	291 (67.2)	315 (61.6)		195 (70.4)	185 (66.8)	
Black	70 (16.2)	62 (12.1)		11 (4.0)	5 (1.8)	
Hispanic	51 (11.8)	91 (17.8)	*	23 (8.3)	18 (6.5)	
Asian/Pacific Islander	...	...	...	32 (11.6)	51 (18.4)	*
Asian, other	...	...	...	14 (5.1)	15 (5.4)	
Other	21 (4.9)	43 (8.4)	*	2 (0.7)	3 (1.1)	
Foreign-born	121 (26.8)	158 (30.3)		59 (21.2)	82 (29.6)	*
Postsecondary education, No. (%)	259 (57.3)	317 (70.0)		266 (95.7)	270 (97.5)	
Children ≤ 18 y in household	211 (46.7)	246 (47.2)		130 (46.8)	139 (50.2)	
Baseline health characteristics						
10-y CRS, %	7.4 ± 8.0	8.1 ± 7.9		10.3 ± 7.9	9.6 ± 7.0	
Systolic blood pressure, mm Hg	114.8 ± 12.3	114.8 ± 13.5		120.2 ± 13.2	117.8 ± 13.5	*
BMI, kg/m^2	29.5 ± 7.0	29.5 ± 6.9		28.7 ± 5.4	28.0 ± 5.7	
HbA_{1c}, %	5.5 ± 0.6	5.5 ± 0.6		5.7 ± 0.6	5.6 ± 0.5	
Smoker	127 (28.1)	154 (29.6)		18 (6.5)	17 (6.1)	
HDL cholesterol, mg/dl	64.1 ± 5.8	63.1 ± 5.3	*	65.3 ± 5.4	64.4 ± 4.7	*
Total cholesterol, mg/dl	191.2 ± 28.9	190.8 ± 28.4		194.3 ± 27.2	190.5 ± 23.0	
12-mo health characteristics						
10-y CRS, %	7.3 ± 7.8	8.3 ± 8.4		10.2 ± 7.8	9.7 ± 7.2	
Systolic blood pressure, mm Hg	111.5 ± 12.0	112.3 ± 13.9		116.8 ± 12.5	115.9 ± 14.0	
BMI, kg/m^2	29.5 ± 6.8	29.8 ± 6.8		28.7 ± 5.6	27.9 ± 5.7	
HbA_{1c}, %	5.4 ± 0.8	5.5 ± 0.7		5.6 ± 0.6	5.6 ± 0.5	
Smoker	109 (24.1)	146 (28.0)		18 (6.5)	15 (5.4)	
HDL cholesterol, mg/dl	62.4 ± 6.1	61.9 ± 5.8		61.3 ± 5.2	61.4 ± 5.5	
Total cholesterol, mg/dl	197.4 ± 28.8	199.5 ± 28.0		201.2 ± 27.7	202.4 ± 23.9	

Note. BMI = body mass index (weight in kilograms divided by square of height in meters); CRS = cardiometabolic risk score; HDL = high-density lipoprotein; IT = information technology industry. Significance (Δ) is from the Mantel-Haenzel χ^2 test if dichotomous and from the *t* test using pooled or Satterthwaite variances, as appropriate. Race/ethnicity was self-reported. Actual sample sizes differ slightly for baseline sociodemographics: n = 944–973 for long-term care and 554–555 for IT.

*Statistically significant ($P < .05$) within industry differences.

DISCUSSION

The Work, Family and Health Study is among the first studies to use a fully randomized and intent-to-treat design to evaluate whether changing workplace conditions will affect employees' cardiovascular risk. Our findings in 2 different industries suggest common effects. Although there were no main effects of the workplace intervention in either industry for CRS, we did observe an intervention effect among those with higher baseline CRS (Figure 2). Intervention effects for those with elevated baseline CRS were on the order of the effects of lower age-related CRS of 5 to 10 years. Among those with a lower

TABLE 2— Multilevel Intervention Effects on Estimated 10-Year CRS by Industry: United States, 2009–2013

	CRS, Mean (95% CI) or B (95% CI)	
	Long-Term Care	IT
CRS: by group and time		
Usual practice, baseline	8.12 (7.25, 8.99)	9.99 (8.57, 11.41)
Usual practice, 12 mo	8.30 (7.43, 9.18)	10.09 (8.68, 11.51)
Intervention, baseline	7.36 (6.45, 8.28)	9.87 (8.29, 11.45)
Intervention, 12 mo	7.27 (6.36, 8.19)	9.77 (8.19, 11.35)
Overall: difference-in-difference models		
Main effect: time (ref = baseline)	0.18 (−0.06, 0.43)	0.10 (−0.18, 0.39)
Main effect: intervention (ref = usual practice)	−0.76 (−2.08, 0.56)	−0.12 (−2.44, 2.21)
2-way interaction: intervention × 12 mo	−0.27 (−0.63, 0.08)	−0.21 (−0.62, 0.20)
Moderation analysis: difference-in-difference models by baseline CRS		
Main effect: time (ref = baseline)	0.18 (−0.06, 0.42)	0.10 (−0.18, 0.39)
Main effect: intervention (ref = usual practice)	0.01 (−0.29, 0.31)	0.09 (−0.29, 0.48)
Main effect: baseline CRS	1.00 (0.98, 1.02)	1.00 (0.97, 1.03)
2-way interaction (12 mo × baseline CRS)	0.00 (−0.03, 0.03)	−0.01 (−0.05, 0.03)
2-way interaction (intervention × baseline CRS)	0.00 (−0.03, 0.03)	−0.00 (−0.04, 0.04)
2-way interaction (intervention × 12 mo)	−0.31 (−0.66, 0.05)	−0.18 (−0.58, 0.22)
3-way interaction (intervention × 12 mo × baseline CRS)	−0.08 (−0.13, −0.04)	−0.07 (−0.12, −0.01)

Note. CI = confidence interval; CRS = cardiometabolic risk score; ICC = intracluster correlation coefficients; IT = information technology industry. Intervention effects on estimated 10-y CRS by industry were calculated using multilevel models, controlling for number of employees in cluster for long-term care and controlling for whether cluster was assigned rather than randomized, number of employees in cluster, the function (core or support) used for randomization, and whether the merger had been announced at the time of the study for IT. Moderation analyses include additional 3-way interactions between time, intervention, and baseline CRS. The sample size was 1946 (973 per time point) for long-term care and 1110 (555 per time point) for IT. Negative values indicate a decrease in CRS. Lastly, ICCs of participants in workgroups were estimated for all 4 models and are reported here (overall: long-term care ICC = 0.016, IT ICC = 0.064; moderation analysis: long-term care ICC = 0.009, IT ICC < 0.001).

baseline CRS (e.g., younger workers), there may have been floor effects, indicating that it would be very challenging to further reduce the CRS. The strong effect of age on the increase in the 10-year hard cardiovascular disease event is well established.[14,32] Thus, the results indicate that the workplace intervention reduced increases in CRS in more vulnerable workers.

Strengths and Limitations

There are a number of issues that may have affected results. First, although we conducted an intention-to-treat analysis including all those with follow-up data, we included employees who completed the baseline survey and either left the workplace or refused to participate in follow-up using values with last observation carried forward, which yielded consistent moderated intervention effects regardless of analytic approach. Our analysis of attritors suggests that they were not differentially lost to follow-up by treatment assignment. Second, as with all intention-to-treat analyses, we included those who did not participate in intervention sessions or did not receive enough intervention in analyses. When only a fraction of employees and supervisors fully participated, this served to dilute any effects.

The use of a summary cardiometabolic score as a primary outcome has both advantages and disadvantages. The advantages are embedded in additive impacts of small changes in risk across each risk factor. As in the Framingham risk factor score, the summary score is a potent and reliable indicator of future cardiometabolic morbidity and mortality. As with the original score, our score is designed to reflect age- and sex-specific risks. The disadvantage of such a summary score is that it does not enable one to see whether selective risk factors responded differentially to the intervention. A major strength of our study was that interviewers were blind to intervention status, and results relied primarily on biomarkers collected and without the researcher knowing which group respondents were in. We validated CRS outcome on the independent Framingham Offspring cohort.[23]

The pathways by which a social intervention such as ours might influence cardiometabolic risk are multiple and include psychosocial mechanisms, biological pathways, and health behaviors. Our intervention did not include a health behavior change component but focused on work conditions hypothesized to be determinants of health. In this model, more proximate factors may directly mediate relationships between a workplace intervention and health outcomes. In previous publications, we reported that the intervention influenced both distress and depressive symptoms and sleep.[33–35]

This study has limitations. The follow-up period was limited to 12 months, which may not be long enough to assess whether the effects of the intervention were sustained. CRS measures

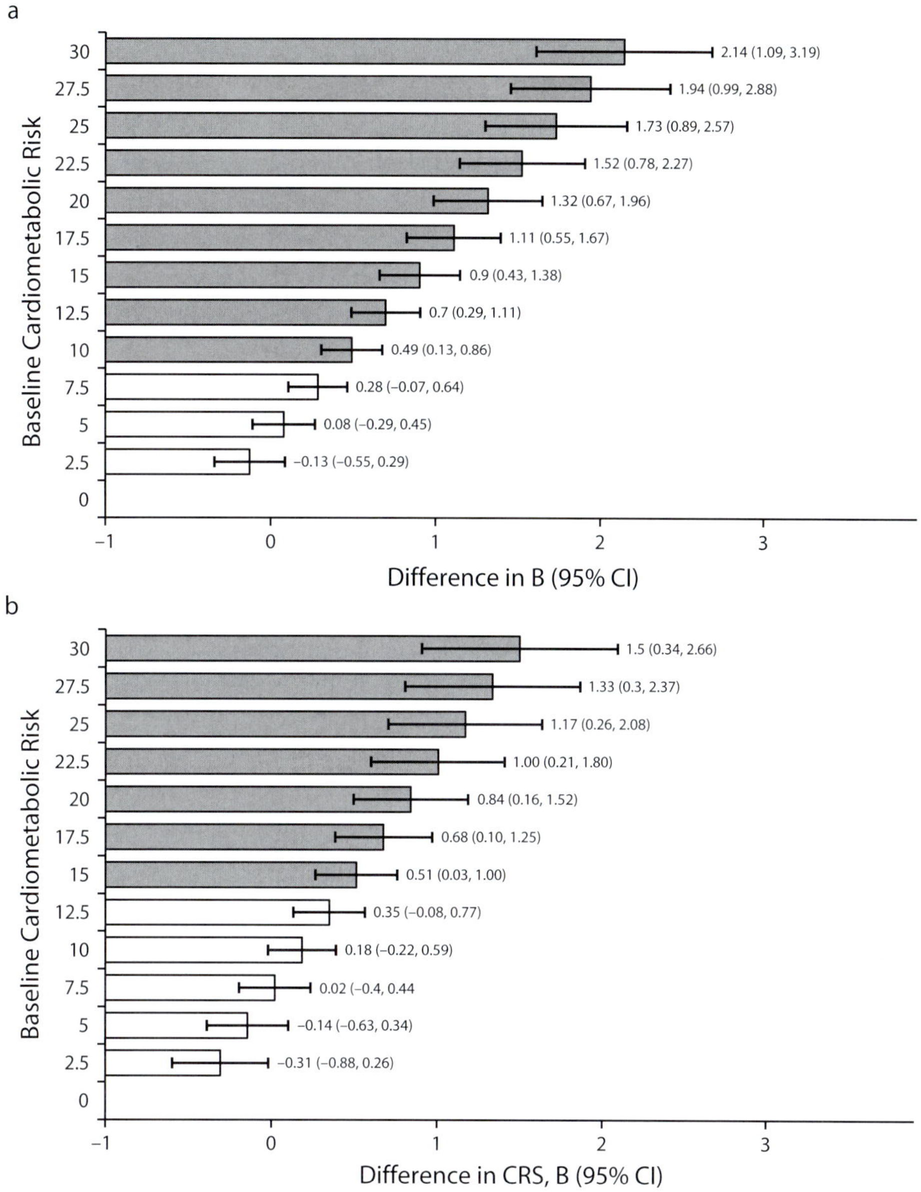

FIGURE 2— **Workplace Intervention Effects on Estimated 10-Year Cardiometabolic Risk Score (CRS) for (a) Long-Term Care Industry Employees and (b) IT Industry Employees: United States, 2009–2013**

Note. CI = confidence interval; CRS = risk of 10-year cardiovascular disease event. Difference in CRS = intervention change minus usual practice change. Shading (darker bars) indicates estimates significantly different from 0 at $P < .05$. Intervention effects on estimated 10-year CRS by industry were calculated using multilevel models, controlling for number of employees in cluster for long-term care and controlling for whether cluster was assigned rather than randomized, number of employees in cluster, the function (core or support) used for randomization, and whether the merger had been announced at the time of the study for IT. The sample size was 1946 (973 per time point) for long-term care and 1110 (555 per time point) for IT. Differences in intervention effects by baseline CRS were statistically significant at $P < .05$. Estimates are shown in Table A (available as a supplement to the online version of this article at http://www.ajph.org).

did not include clinical evaluation or medical records. Although the study included employees from numerous locations in 2 industries, future studies are needed to improve generalizability. Of note, we developed the sex-specific CRS algorithms[36] we used as the outcome with a cohort that was predominately non-Hispanic White. Given that at least 30% of our study participants were of races/ethnicities other than non-Hispanic White, there is a potential risk to validity. However, if there is bias or measurement error, the randomization balanced the proportion of race/ethnicity by intervention groups, and the findings should be relatively unaffected by this error. Nevertheless, future studies should consider recalibrated measures of the CRS for other racial/ethnic groups.[37]

Conclusions

Few randomized trials have been conducted to assess whether changing the work environment can affect cardiovascular risk. Ours is among the first of the trials to do so. In light of recent findings reporting weak or null effects of workplace wellness programs,[7,38] it is important to identify work conditions per se that may affect employee health. Our goal was to change workplace conditions we hypothesized were influencing employee health rather than ask employees to adapt to stressful working conditions via programs that did not change the environment. Our findings suggest that older workers and those with higher cardiovascular risk will benefit from such interventions. We followed a social determinants of health framework reviewed in earlier work in *AJPH*,[8] and we emphasize the need to conduct well-designed experimental workplace redesign interventions aimed at improving health and well-being. Earlier work from the WFHN reported effects on psychological distress, sleep, and a number of safety and organizational behaviors. To our knowledge, this is the first to report the impact on cardiometabolic risk.

Our findings align with much recent work identifying health risks related to low schedule control, long work hours, and lean or just-in-time operations, especially for low- and middle-wage earners.[39] Flexible work policies and practices were increasingly seen during the COVID-19 pandemic as essential for maintaining worker health as well as the health of family and community members. Our findings support the direct impact of workplace organization on the health of workers. AJPH

ABOUT THE AUTHORS

Lisa F. Berkman is with the Harvard Center for Population and Development Studies, Cambridge, MA. Erin L. Kelly is with the Massachusetts Institute of Technology Sloan School of Management, Cambridge. Leslie B. Hammer is with the Center for Occupational Health Sciences, Oregon Health Sciences University, Portland. Frank Mierzwa is with RTI International, Research Triangle Park, NC. Todd Bodner is with the Department of Psychology, Portland State University, Portland, OR. Tay McNamara is with the Women's Studies Research Center, Brandeis University, Waltham, MA. Hayami K. Koga is with the Department of Social and Behavioral Sciences, Harvard T. H. Chan School of Public Health, Boston, MA. Soomi Lee is with the Department of Human Development and Family Studies, Pennsylvania State University, University Park. Miguel Marino is with the Department of Family Medicine, Oregon Health & Science University, Portland. Laura C. Klein and Orfeu M. Buxton are with the Department of Biobehavioral Health, Pennsylvania State University, University Park. Thomas W. McDade is with the Department of Anthropology, Northwestern University, Evanston, IL. Ginger Hanson is with the Johns Hopkins School of Nursing, Baltimore, MD. Phyllis Moen is with the Department of Sociology, University of Minnesota, Minneapolis.

CORRESPONDENCE

Correspondence should be sent to Lisa F. Berkman, 9 Bow St, Cambridge, MA 02138 (e-mail: lberkman@hsph.harvard.edu). Reprints can be ordered at http://www.ajph.org by clicking the "Reprints" link.

PUBLICATION INFORMATION

Full Citation: Berkman LF, Kelly EL, Hammer LB, et al. Employee cardiometabolic risk following a cluster-randomized workplace intervention from the Work, Family and Health Network, 2009–2013. *Am J Public Health*. 2023;113(12):1322–1331.

Acceptance Date: August 13, 2023.

DOI: http://doi.org/10.2105/AJPH.2023.307413

CONTRIBUTORS

L. F. Berkman, E. L. Kelly, L. B. Hammer, F. Mierzwa, T. Bodner, M. Marino, L. C. Klein, T. W. McDade, G. Hanson, P. Moen, and O. M. Buxton were involved in original data collection and analysis and writing the article. T. McNamara, H. K. Koga, and S. Lee were instrumental in statistical analysis and writing the article.

ACKNOWLEDGMENTS

This research was conducted as part of the Work, Family and Health Network (https://workfamilyhealthnetwork.org), which is funded by a cooperative agreement through the National Institutes of Health (NIH) and the Centers for Disease Control and Prevention: Eunice Kennedy Shriver National Institute of Child Health and Human Development (grants U01HD051217, U01HD051218, U01HD051256, U01HD051276), National Institute on Aging (grant U01AG027669), Office of Behavioral and Social Sciences Research, and National Institute for Occupational Safety and Health (grants U01OH008788, U01HD059773), and the National Heart Lung and Blood Institute (grant R01-HL107240). Grants from the University of Minnesota's College of Liberal Arts, McKnight Foundation, William T. Grant Foundation, Alfred P. Sloan Foundation, and the Administration for Children and Families provided additional funding.

Note. The contents of this publication are solely the responsibility of the authors and do not necessarily represent the official views of any of these institutions or offices.

CONFLICTS OF INTEREST

Outside this work, O. M. Buxton discloses that he received subcontract grants to Pennsylvania State University from Proactive Life (formerly Mobile Sleep Technologies), doing business as SleepSpace (National Science Foundation grant 1622766 and NIH/National Institute on Aging Small Business Innovation Research Program grants R43AG056250, R44 AG056250), received honoraria and travel support for lectures from Boston University, Boston College, Tufts School of Dental Medicine, New York University, University of Miami, University of South Florida, University of Utah, University of Arizona, Harvard T.H. Chan School of Public Health, Eric H. Angle Society of Orthodontists, and Allstate, and consulting fees for SleepNumber. He receives an honorarium for his role as the editor-in-chief of the journal *Sleep Health*.

All other authors have no conflicts of interest to disclose.

HUMAN PARTICIPANT PROTECTION

Study methods were approved by the Harvard T.H. Chan School of Public Health institutional review board (IRB) and the IRBs of other study centers and was conducted in accordance with the Declaration of Helsinki. All participants provided written informed consent before randomization.

REFERENCES

1. Kossek EE, Perrigino M, Rock AG. From ideal workers to ideal work for all: a 50-year review integrating careers and work–family research with a future research agenda. *J Vocat Behav*. 2021;126:103504. https://doi.org/10.1016/j.jvb.2020.103504
2. Nomaguchi KM. Change in work–family conflict among employed parents between 1977 and 1997. *J Marriage Fam*. 2009;71(1):15–32. https://doi.org/10.1111/j.1741-3737.2008.00577.x
3. Winslow S. Work–family conflict, gender, and parenthood, 1977–1997. *J Fam Issues*. 2005;26(6):727–755. https://doi.org/10.1177/0192513X05277522
4. Schieman S, Glavin P, Milkie MA. When work interferes with life: work–nonwork interference and the influence of work-related demands and resources. *Am Sociol Rev*. 2009;74(6):966–988. https://doi.org/10.1177/000312240907400606

5. Jones D, Molitor D, Reif J. What do workplace wellness programs do? Evidence from the Illinois Workplace Wellness Study. *Q J Econ.* 2019;134(4): 1747–1791. https://doi.org/10.1093/qje/qjz023
6. Reif J, Chan D, Jones D, Payne L, Molitor D. Effects of a workplace wellness program on employee health, health beliefs, and medical use: a randomized clinical trial. *JAMA Intern Med.* 2020;180(7): 952–960. https://doi.org/10.1001/jamainternmed.2020.1321
7. Song Z, Baicker K. Effect of a workplace wellness program on employee health and economic outcomes: a randomized clinical trial. *JAMA.* 2019; 321(15):1491–1501. https://doi.org/10.1001/jama.2019.3307
8. Lovejoy M, Kelly EL, Kubzansky LD, Berkman LF. Work redesign for the 21st century: promising strategies for enhancing worker well-being. *Am J Public Health.* 2021;111(10):1787–1795. https://doi.org/10.2105/AJPH.2021.306283
9. Fox KE, Johnson ST, Berkman LF, et al. Organisational- and group-level workplace interventions and their effect on multiple domains of worker well-being: a systematic review. *Work Stress.* 2022; 36(1):30–59. https://doi.org/10.1080/02678373.2021.1969476
10. Choi B, Schnall P, Ko S, Dobson M, Baker D. Job strain and coronary heart disease. *Lancet.* 2013;381(9865):448. https://doi.org/10.1016/S0140-6736(13)60243-3
11. Kivimäki M, Nyberg ST, Batty GD, et al. Job strain as a risk factor for coronary heart disease: a collaborative meta-analysis of individual participant data. *Lancet.* 2012;380(9852):1491–1497. https://doi.org/10.1016/S0140-6736(12)60994-5
12. Landsbergis P, Schnall P. Job strain and coronary heart disease. *Lancet.* 2013;381(9865):448. [Comment in: Kivimäki M, Singh-Manoux A, Nyberg S, Batty GD. Job strain and coronary heart disease—authors' reply. *Lancet.* 2013;381(9865):448–449. https://doi.org/10.1016/S0140-6736(13)60244-5]. https://doi.org/10.1016/S0140-6736(13)60242-1
13. Sara JD, Prasad M, Eleid MF, Zhang M, Widmer RJ, Lerman A. Association between work-related stress and coronary heart disease: a review of prospective studies through the job strain, effort–reward balance, and organizational justice models. *J Am Heart Assoc.* 2018;7(9):e008073. https://doi.org/10.1161/JAHA.117.008073
14. Berkman LF, Liu SY, Hammer L, et al. Work–family conflict, cardiometabolic risk, and sleep duration in nursing employees. *J Occup Health Psychol.* 2015;20(4):420–433. https://doi.org/10.1037/a0039143
15. Hammer LB, Sauter S. Total worker health and work–life stress. 2013;55(12, suppl):S25–S29. https://doi.org/10.1097/JOM.0000000000000043
16. Lloyd Jones DM, Allen NB, Anderson CAM, et al. Life's essential 8: updating and enhancing the American Heart Association's construct of cardiovascular health: a presidential advisory from the American Heart Association. *Circulation.* 2022; 146(5):e18–e43. https://doi.org/10.1161/CIR.0000000000001078
17. Amiri S, Behnezhad S. Association between job strain and sick leave: a systematic review and meta-analysis of prospective cohort studies. *Public Health.* 2020;185:235–242. https://doi.org/10.1016/j.puhe.2020.05.023
18. Ertel KA, Berkman LF, Buxton OM. Socioeconomic status, occupational characteristics, and sleep duration in African/Caribbean immigrants and US White health care workers. *Sleep.* 2011;34(4): 509–518. https://doi.org/10.1093/sleep/34.4.509
19. Kivimäki M, Kawachi I. Work stress as a risk factor for cardiovascular disease. *Curr Cardiol Rep.* 2015; 17(9):630. https://doi.org/10.1007/s11886-015-0630-8
20. Brossoit RM, Crain TL, Hammer LB, Lee S, Bodner TE, Buxton OM. Associations among patient care workers' schedule control, sleep, job satisfaction and turnover intentions. *Stress Health.* 2020;36(4):442–456. https://doi.org/10.1002/smi.2941
21. Kelly EL, Moen P, Oakes JM, et al. Changing work and work–family conflict: evidence from the work, family, and health network. *Am Sociol Rev.* 2014;79(3):485–516. https://doi.org/10.1177/0003122414531435
22. Kossek EE, Hammer LB, Kelly EL, Moen P. Designing work, family & health organizational change initiatives. *Organ Dyn.* 2014;43(1):53–63. https://doi.org/10.1016/j.orgdyn.2013.10.007
23. Marino M, Li Y, Pencina MJ, D'Agostino RB Sr, Berkman LF, Buxton OM. Quantifying cardiometabolic risk using modifiable non-self-reported risk factors. *Am J Prev Med.* 2014;47(2):131–140. https://doi.org/10.1016/j.amepre.2014.03.006
24. Uchino BN, Berg CA, Smith TW, Pearce G, Skinner M. Age-related differences in ambulatory blood pressure during daily stress: evidence for greater blood pressure reactivity with age. *Psychol Aging.* 2006;21(2):231–239. https://doi.org/10.1037/0882-7974.21.2.231
25. Winning A, Glymour MM, McCormick MC, Gilsanz P, Kubzansky LD. Psychological distress across the life course and cardiometabolic risk. *J Am Coll Cardiol.* 2015;66(14):1577–1586. https://doi.org/10.1016/j.jacc.2015.08.021
26. Bray JW, Kelly EL, Hammer LB, et al. *An integrative, multilevel, and transdisciplinary research approach to challenges of work, family, and health.* Research Triangle Park, NC: RTI Press; 2013. https://doi.org/10.3768/rtipress.2013.mr.0024.1303
27. Frane JW. A method of biased coin randomization, its implementation, and its validation. *Ther Innov Regul Sci.* 1998;32:423–432. https://doi.org/10.1177/009286159803200213
28. Berkman LF, Buxton OM, Ertel K, Okechukwu C. Manager's practices related to work–family balance predict employee cardiovascular risk and sleep duration in extended care settings. *J Occup Health Psychol.* 2010;15(3):316–329. https://doi.org/10.1037/a0019721
29. Moen P, Kelly EL, Tranby E, Huang Q. Changing work, changing health: can real work-time flexibility promote health behaviors and well-being? *J Health Soc Behav.* 2011;52(4):404–429. https://doi.org/10.1177/0022146511418979
30. Hammer LB, Truxillo DM, Bodner T, Rineer J, Pytlovany AC, Richman A. Effects of a workplace intervention targeting psychosocial risk factors on safety and health outcomes. *BioMed Res Int.* 2015;2015:836967. https://doi.org/10.1155/2015/836967
31. Samuelsson LB, Hall MH, McLean S, et al. Validation of biomarkers of CVD risk from dried blood spots in community-based research: methodologies and study-specific serum equivalencies. *Biodemography Soc Biol.* 2015;61(3):285–297. https://doi.org/10.1080/19485565.2015.1068105
32. Buxton OM, Lee S, Marino M, Beverly C, Almeida DM, Berkman L. Sleep health and predicted cardiometabolic risk scores in employed adults from two industries. *J Clin Sleep Med.* 2018;14(3): 371–383. https://doi.org/10.5664/jcsm.6980
33. Lee S, Almeida DM, Berkman L, Olson R, Moen P, Buxton OM. Age differences in workplace intervention effects on employees' nighttime and daytime sleep. *Sleep Health.* 2016;2(4):289–296. https://doi.org/10.1016/j.sleh.2016.08.004
34. Olson R, Crain TL, Bodner TE, et al. A workplace intervention improves sleep: results from the randomized controlled work, family, and health study. *Sleep Health.* 2015;1(1):55–65. https://doi.org/10.1016/j.sleh.2014.11.003
35. Kossek EE, Thompson RJ, Lawson KM, et al. Caring for the elderly at work and home: can a randomized organizational intervention improve psychological health? *J Occup Health Psychol.* 2019;24(1):36–54. https://doi.org/10.1037/ocp0000104
36. Marino M, Li Y, Pencina MJ, D'Agostino RB, Berkman LF, Buxton OM. Quantifying cardiometabolic risk using modifiable non-self-reported risk factors. *Am J Prev Med.* 2014;47(2):131–140. https://doi.org/10.1016/j.amepre.2014.03.006
37. D'Agostino RB Sr, Grundy S, Sullivan LM, Wilson P; CHD Risk Prediction Group. Validation of the Framingham coronary heart disease prediction scores: results of a multiple ethnic groups investigation. *JAMA.* 2001;286(2):180–187. https://doi.org/10.1001/jama.286.2.180
38. Jones D, Molitor D, Reif J. *What Do Workplace Wellness Programs Do? Evidence From the Illinois Workplace Wellness Study.* Cambridge, MA: National Bureau of Economic Research; 2018. NBER working paper 24229. https://doi.org/10.3386/w24229
39. Kelly EL, Moen P. *Overload: How Good Jobs Went Bad and What We Can Do About It.* Princeton, NJ: Princeton University Press; 2020. https://doi.org/10.1515/9780691200033

Health Effects of High-Concentration Cannabis Products: Scoping Review and Evidence Map

Lisa Bero, PhD, Rosa Lawrence, BA, Jean-Pierre Oberste, BA, Tianjing Li, MD, PhD, MHS, Louis Leslie, BA, Thanitsara Rittiphairoj, MD, MPH, Christi Piper, MLIS, George Sam Wang, MD, Ashley Brooks-Russell, PhD, MPH, Tsz Wing Yim, MPH, Gregory Tung, PhD, MPH, and Jonathan M. Samet, MD, MS

Background. The concentration of pharmacologically active tetrahydrocannabinol (THC) in cannabis products has been increasing over the past decade. Concerns about potential harmful health effects of using these increasingly higher-concentration products have led some states to consider regulation of cannabis product THC concentration. We conducted a scoping review of health effects of high-concentration cannabis products to inform policy on whether the THC concentrations of cannabis product should be regulated or limited.

Objectives. We conducted a scoping review to (1) identify and describe human studies that explore the relationship of high-concentration cannabis products with any health outcomes in the literature and (2) create an interactive evidence map of the included studies to facilitate further analyses.

Search Methods. An experienced medical information specialist designed a comprehensive search strategy of 7 electronic databases.

Selection Criteria. We included human studies of any epidemiological design with no restrictions by age, sex, health status, country, or outcome measured that reported THC concentration or included a known high-concentration cannabis product.

Data Collection and Analysis. We imported search results into Distiller SR, and trained coders conducted artificial intelligence–assisted screening. We developed, piloted, and revised data abstraction forms. One person performed data abstraction, and a senior reviewer verified a subset. We provide a tabular description of study characteristics, including exposures and outcomes measured, for each included study. We interrogated the evidence map published in Tableau to answer specific questions and provide the results as text and visual displays.

Main Results. We included 452 studies in the scoping review and evidence map. There was incomplete reporting of exposure characteristics including THC concentration, duration and frequency of use, and products used. The evidence map shows considerable heterogeneity among studies in exposures, outcomes, and populations studied. A limited number of reports provided data that would facilitate further quantitative synthesis of the results across studies.

Conclusions. This scoping review and evidence map support strong conclusions concerning the utility of the literature for characterizing risks and benefits of the current cannabis marketplace and the research approaches followed in the studies identified. Relevance of the studies to today's products is limited.

Public Health Implications. High-quality evidence to address the policy question of whether the THC concentration of cannabis products should be regulated is scarce. The publicly available interactive evidence map is a timely resource for other entities concerned with burgeoning access to high-concentration cannabis. (*Am J Public Health.* 2023;113(12):1332–1342. https://doi.org/10.2105/AJPH.2023.307414)

AJPH December 2023, Vol 113, No. 12

PLAIN-LANGUAGE SUMMARY

The potency or tetrahydrocannabinol (THC) concentration in cannabis products has been increasing over the past decade. Policymakers have become interested in whether THC concentration should be regulated. To inform these discussions, we conducted a scoping review and created an evidence map of human studies that explore the relationship of high-concentration cannabis products with any health outcomes. The evidence map including 452 studies shows considerable variability in exposures, outcomes, and populations studied. A limited number of reports provided data that would facilitate synthesis of the results across studies. High-quality evidence to address the policy question of whether the THC concentration of cannabis products should be regulated is scarce. The publicly available interactive evidence map is a timely resource for policymakers and researchers concerned about the increasing access to high-concentration cannabis.

The concentration of pharmacologically active tetrahydrocannabinol (THC) in cannabis products has been increasing over the past decade. While smoking of cannabis products has been declining, routes of administration that use higher-concentration THC products, such as vaping and dabbing, have been increasing.[1,2] Concerns about potential harmful health effects of using these high-concentration products and these routes of administration have also been on the rise.[3–6]

As of February 2023, 37 states allowed medical cannabis, and 19 states had legalized recreational cannabis, providing access to high-concentration products.[7,8] Because of growing use of high-concentration products and related health concerns, several states including Connecticut, Illinois, New York, and Washington, have begun to regulate cannabis product "potency," defined as THC concentration. The rationale for such regulation is that high-concentration cannabis products may pose a greater risk of harmful health effects than lower-concentration products. Colorado House Bill 21-1317 (HB 1317; Concerning the Regulation of Marijuana for Safe Consumption, and, in Connection Therewith, Making an Appropriation) required the Colorado School of Public Health to "do a systematic review of the scientific research related to the physical and mental health effects of high-potency THC marijuana and concentrates."[9] The review has high public health relevancy because the Colorado state legislature commissioned it to inform policy on whether the THC concentration of cannabis product should be regulated or limited. The review team was tasked to cover both harmful and beneficial health outcomes, but the completed review is not focused on clinical uses of cannabis.

The broad question posed by the Colorado state legislature was ideally suited to a scoping review approach. A scoping review is performed to map key concepts, types of evidence, and gaps in research related to a defined area or field.[10] Given the heterogeneity in how concentration of cannabis is defined, the broad range of outcomes of interest, and the variety of study designs used to study the health effects of high-concentration cannabis products, the scoping review aimed to clarify the key concepts related to how high concentration is defined, examine how research on harms and benefits of cannabis is conducted, describe the key characteristics associated with these studies, and identify gaps in the evidence.[11] Because scoping reviews use systematic review methods, we also aimed to identify subsets of homogeneous studies potentially eligible for future synthesis.

Evidence maps refer to a wide range of practices that visually display evidence synthesis products. Evidence maps are increasingly used, particularly in environmental health, to display the results of scoping reviews of animal and human evidence.[12,13] The aim of an evidence map is to catalog and describe evidence rather than to synthesize findings. An evidence map provides an interactive, user-friendly searchable database or visual display of systematically identified literature on a given topic.[14,15] By giving a picture of the scope of evidence available, it is a public health good for a broad range of users. An evidence map can be used to identify studies with certain common characteristics, such as outcomes and exposures studied. Users can also interrogate the map to identify studies that can answer a particular policy question and possibly conduct a full systematic review and meta-analysis.[12]

We describe the scoping review on high-concentration cannabis with the dual goals of documenting the utility of this approach to evidence identification and introducing the evidence map to the public health community.

The objectives of the scoping review were to (1) identify and describe human studies that explore the relationship of high-concentration cannabis products with any health outcomes and (2) create an interactive evidence map of included studies to facilitate further analysis.

METHODS

Details on the methods can be found in the published protocol for this scoping review.[16] R. L., J.-P. O., and T. W. K. were added as authors because of their contributions following publication of the protocol. We used Joanna Briggs Institute[17] and Cochrane[18] methodologies for conducting scoping reviews.

Study Selection Criteria

We included research conducted in any country on recreational (nonprescription) cannabis use, medicinal cannabis use, or both. We included studies conducted in humans of any age and excluded animal studies, as well as laboratory or simulation-based mechanistic studies. We included studies of any epidemiological design.

THC concentration of products. We included studies that reported THC concentration for a cannabis product taken by any route or that reported a product description (e.g., "high-potency concentrate," "dab," and other names for concentrates) from which a high concentration could be inferred.

THC concentration is not the same as dose or level of exposure. Dose refers to the potential amount of THC available to the consumer of the product. The physiologic effect or health outcome experienced is influenced by THC concentration, the specific type of cannabis product, route of administration, duration of use, frequency of use, experience or tolerance of the user and their ability to self-titrate. Therefore, we included studies that assessed a dose–response relationship or supported reaching a conclusion about dose.

We included reports that measured THC concentration in different ways (e.g., percentage THC, mg THC).

Some analyses of cannabis health effects use a THC:cannabidiol (CBD) ratio for medicinal use. Products with a high THC:CBD ratio may have a relatively low concentration of THC. Thus, we excluded studies that reported a THC:CBD ratio only and no THC concentration.

Types of products. We included exposures to the following types of cannabis products: plant (dried or undried), edibles, oral capsule or pill preparation, concentrated extract, oils, tinctures, marijuana e-cigarettes, and other or unknown preparations. We excluded CBD or cannabinol-only products and studies of dronabinol, nabilone, and other orally administered medicinal synthetic cannabinoid products.

Health outcomes. We included any health outcomes studied regardless of whether classified as beneficial or adverse. We extracted the verbatim text for each outcome and categorized each according to previous authoritative reports on cannabis.[3–5] Categories were mental health, neurologic, pain, cardiometabolic, gastrointestinal, psychosocial, sleep, substance use or dependence, respiratory, cancer, ocular, injury and death, immunity, sexual and reproductive health, pregnancy-related outcomes (mother), and pre-, peri-, and neonatal outcomes.

Data Sources and Searches

A medical information specialist (C. P.) designed and conducted a comprehensive search for the concepts of marijuana or THC. Relevant publications were identified by searching 7 databases with a combination of controlled vocabulary and keywords. We limited the searches to English language and human studies. We excluded comments, editorials, interviews, news articles, and letters as publication types. We did not apply any date limitation. The search strategy was peer-reviewed by another medical information specialist before execution using the PRESS checklist[10] (see "Search Strategy and Number of Records Identified" in the Appendix, available as a supplement to the online version of this article at https://ajph.org). We conducted the initial search in October 2021 and updated it in July 2022. We exported all results to DistillerSR[19] where duplicates were identified and removed automatically.

Study Selection

Title and abstract screening. We used the artificial intelligence (AI) text-mining features available in DistillerSR to assist in screening.[19] We trained the AI screening prioritization algorithm using 1000 randomly selected records. These records were screened and labeled by 2 senior screeners (L. L., T. R.) coding independently, with discrepancies decided by discussion (T. L., L. B., L. L., T. R.).

We used the "trained" DistillerSR's AI algorithm to rank the remaining unreviewed titles and abstracts. This set of references used continuous AI prioritization; with every 200 records screened, the AI algorithm ranks and reorders records so those scored highly for inclusion are screened sooner.

Full-text screening. We retrieved full-text reports of potentially relevant citations. Two screeners (combinations of L. L., J.-P. O., T. R., T. W. Y., and trained graduate students) reviewed the full text against the eligibility criteria independently with disagreements decided by a senior review team member (L. B. or T. L.). Reasons for excluding full-text reports were recorded.

Quality control and quality assurance. Two reviewers (L. L. and T. R.) checked 2% of all screening decisions at both titles and abstracts and full text screening stages, discussed problems at routine group meetings, and retrained screeners as needed. We also ran the DistillerSRs "Check for Screening Errors" tool to check the human screening decisions against the AI rankings.[19] A senior reviewer (L. L. or T. R.) reevaluated flagged references for inclusion.

We report the search and selection according to the Preferred Reporting Items for Systematic Reviews and Meta-analyses extension for scoping reviews (PRISMA-ScR).[20] No reviewers involved in screening have published research on cannabis that could be eligible for inclusion and, therefore, they did not have an a priori basis to introduce bias in the selection of studies.

Data Collection

We developed and pilot tested a data extraction form in DistillerSR to manually extract study details from full-text reports. One reviewer extracted data into the data extraction form, which was checked by senior reviewers (L. L., J.-P. O., T. R., T. W. Y.). We extracted data on the following:

- publication information, including authors, type of report, journal, year, type of publication, funding source, country;
- study topic and objectives;
- study design, including location, setting, and inclusion and exclusion criteria;
- characteristics of population, including age, developmental stage, sex, race/ethnicity, indicators of health equity, pregnancy status, and comorbidities;
- details of exposure, including type of cannabis product, route of administration, duration, frequency of intake, experience or tolerance of user, self-titration, and concentration;
- details of comparison exposure, if applicable; and
- outcomes, including outcome domain, outcome descriptor, measurement method, metric, method of aggregation, and time point.

The complete list of data extraction items can be found at our Open Science Framework Project page: https://osf.io/9kndw/?view_only=b6f472d680af41bc84e8a6aa337fd04b.

As per scoping review methods, we did not assess risk of bias for primary studies because of heterogeneity of study designs included.[21]

Presentation and Analysis of Included Studies

To facilitate exploration of the extracted information from the scoping review and to provide a resource to other researchers and the public, we created a publicly available evidence map. All extracted data were exported from DistillerSR to R Studio and reformatted into multiple data sets for the evidence map in Tableau. We used study ID to link all evidence map components, enabling cross-filtering. The evidence map is published to the University of Colorado public Tableau server:

https://viz-public.cu.edu/#/site/Anschutz/views/EvidenceMap/Home?:iid=1.

We provide a tabular description of study characteristics, including exposures and outcomes measured, for each included study.

We interrogated the evidence map to address the following questions, relevant to current policy discussions, and provide the results as text and visual displays:

- Of the different types of cannabis products studied, how many have reported THC concentration, frequency, or duration?
- What THC concentrations have been reported in the literature?
- What types of outcomes have been examined for studies that reported THC concentration?
- What types of outcomes have been studied for the different types of cannabis products?
- What THC concentrations have been studied by outcome?

RESULTS

Database searches identified 49 729 unique titles and abstracts for screening, resulting in 5828 full text reports. We included 452 studies in the scoping review (367 observational studies or randomized trials and 85 case reports or case series) and evidence map (Figure 1). The earliest publication date of an included study was 1971, and 60% (n = 269) of the studies were published between 2017 and 2022.

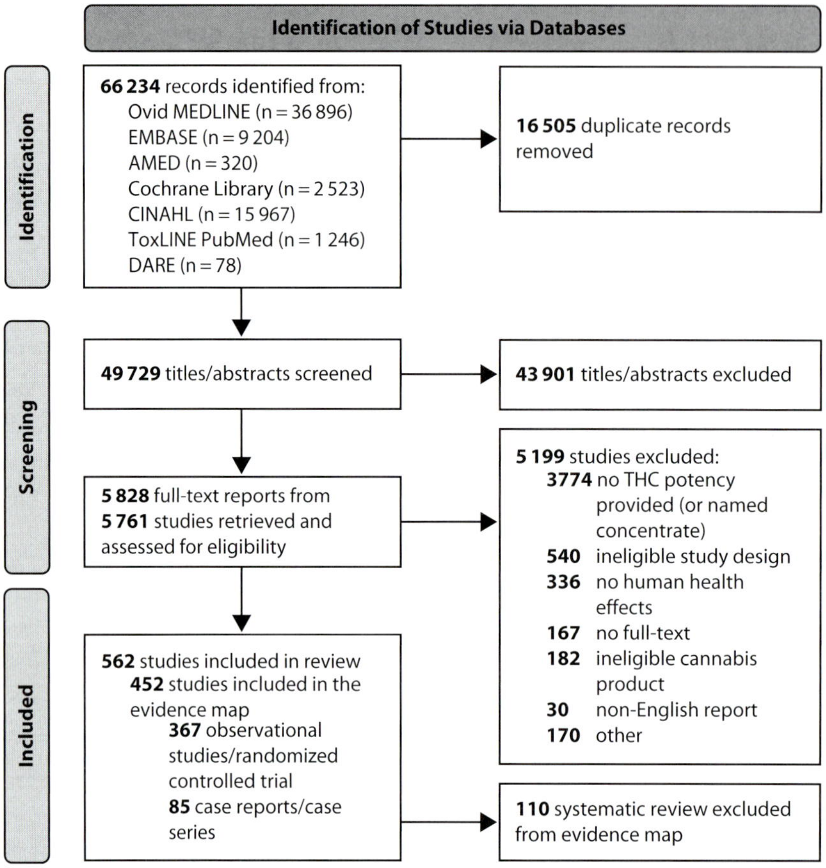

FIGURE 1— PRISMA Diagram for Study Identification for Health Effects of High-Concentration Cannabis Products: Scoping Review and Evidence Map

Note. PRISMA = Preferred Reporting Items for Systematic Reviews and Meta-analyses; THC = tetrahydrocannabinol.

Evidence Map

The interactive evidence map is available at https://viz-public.cu.edu/#/site/Anschutz/views/EvidenceMap/Home?:iid=1.

Bibliographic details for the 452 included studies are provided in the evidence map. The dashboard is organized so that studies can be sorted by study characteristics, population investigated, exposures to cannabis products, and health outcomes. The dashboard links to bibliographic information and the abstracts for all studies identified.

Characteristics of Included Studies

The characteristics of included studies are summarized in Appendix Table A. The 452 studies had variable objectives: harm of a product (n = 349; 77%) and efficacy for a therapeutic indication (n = 233; 52%). Cannabis products addressed in the studies were used for several reasons including medicinal use (n = 177; 39%), recreational use (n = 68; 15%), and unintentional use (n = 20; 4%). One hundred fifty-six studies reported some other purpose of cannabis use (35%), and 87 studies did not report the purpose of cannabis use (19%).

The studies were classified by study design: observational studies (n = 225; 50%), randomized control trials (n = 142; 31%), case reports (n = 51; 11%), and case series (n = 34; 8%).

The studies were conducted across multiple countries, primarily in the United States (n = 220; 49%), the United Kingdom (n = 46; 10%), and Canada (n = 45; 10%). There was at least 1 study from 27 other countries. Within the United States, studies were done primarily in California (n = 47; 10%), Colorado (n = 27; 6%), and New York (n = 18; 4%), but participants from all states other than Alabama, Delaware, and West Virginia were involved in at least 1 study.

Disclosures of study funding source, author affiliations, and conflicts of interest were often lacking: 24% (n = 109) of studies did not report funding source, and 32% (n = 143) of studies did not report if authors had conflicts of interest. A small proportion of studies (n = 25; 6%) were funded by the cannabis industry; 13% (n = 58) had at least 1 author who disclosed a financial tie with the industry.

Only 11% (n = 48) of studies included any analysis on a health equity measure. Less than one tenth of studies (n = 41; 9%) included analysis or stratification by health equity subgroups, 1% (n = 6) of studies focused exclusively on historically excluded populations, and no studies included specific analyses of structural racism or inequalities.

The study populations were variable, including ages from newborn to adults aged older than 65 years, with a range of racial and ethnic groups. Some studies also had restrictions on eligibility requirements, such as a preexisting disease or condition.

Exposures

The most common cannabis products studies were of generic cannabis types (n = 284; 63%). Products that are typically high concentration, such as oils, concentrates, hash, extracts, skunk, and resins, were examined in approximately 2% to 10% of all studies. Overall, 384 studies (85%) reported the frequency of intake, with the most common being daily (n = 177; 39%), and 371 (82%) reported the duration of intake. The route of administration was reported in 393 studies (87%) including inhalation (n = 279; 62%), ingestion (n = 174; 38%), sublingual (n = 39; 9%), and topical (n = 31; 7%).

Studies did not consistently provide complete information on exposure characteristics such as THC concentration and frequency and duration of exposure. Figure 2 addresses the question, "Of the different types of cannabis products studied, how many have reported THC concentration, frequency, or duration?" Details of cannabis exposure were reported most often in studies that included generic cannabis (Figure 2).

There was substantial variability in reporting of THC concentration, including the units and indices used (e.g., range, threshold, exact values, mean). When THC concentration was reported, it was most commonly as percentage of THC (n = 172; 38%) or milligrams of THC (n = 113; 25%). We interrogated the evidence map to address the question, "What THC concentrations have been reported in the literature?" There were 172 studies that reported THC concentration with percentage of THC corresponding to 349 different exposures. For these studies, the median concentration was 12% (mean = 17.4%; range = 0%–100%; Q1 = 3.6%; Q3 = 24%). Of 113 studies with 143 exposures reporting concentration in milligrams of THC, the median concentration was 15 milligrams (mean = 37.4 mg; range = 0.3–500 mg; Q1 = 7. 5 mg; Q3 = 26 mg).

Exposure Reported \ Product Type	Cannabis	Concentrate	Oil	Extract	Skunk	Hash/hashish	Resin	Kief	Dab	Wax	Unspecified	Other
THC concentration	202	17	33	17	3	6	4	0	2	0	53	56
Frequency	246	28	35	17	12	27	8	2	9	3	45	59
Duration	241	29	36	17	11	30	9	2	8	3	40	62

FIGURE 2— Number of Studies With Reported THC Concentration, Frequency, or Duration of Cannabis Use by Cannabis Product Type in Health Effects of High-Concentration Cannabis Products: Scoping Review and Evidence Map

Note. THC = tetrahydrocannabinol. Counts indicate the number of studies with an included cannabis product type and cannabis exposure characteristic. Studies may include multiple product types and exposures. Color saturation indicates the number of studies with a reported product or exposure in relation to other product or exposures. Total n = 446 because 6 studies reported that they tested a high-concentration product but did not report numeric THC concentration, frequency, or duration.

Outcomes

The most common outcome domain for the 452 included studies was mental health (n = 180; 40%), followed by neurologic (n = 134; 30%), pain (n = 133; 29%), cardiometabolic (n = 110; 24%), gastrointestinal (n = 101; 22%), psychosocial (n = 98; 22%), and sleep (n = 94; 21%). Outcome domains are broad. For example, the mental health outcome domain included depression, psychosis, memory, and cognition. Even a single outcome (such as depression) was measured in different ways in different studies (such as depression scales, clinical chart review, or self-report).

We interrogated the evidence map to address the question, "What types of outcomes have been studied for the different types of cannabis products?" We found that the outcome domains studied by product type showed a similar distribution to outcomes studied overall as shown in Appendix Table A.

Studies across all outcome domains reported numeric THC concentrations. Figure 3 addresses the question "What THC concentrations have been studied for the different outcome domains?" Median THC concentrations reported were less than 50 milligrams or 25% THC for all outcome domains studied.

Potential for Evidence Synthesis

Few studies provided data that would facilitate further quantitative synthesis of the results across studies. Fifty-four studies (12%) examined a direct association between cannabis concentrates and a health outcome, whereas 189 (42%) examined a direct association between THC concentration and a health outcome. One hundred fourteen studies (25%) examined an indirect association between THC concentration and health outcomes. Sixty-two studies (14%) examined an indirect association between concentrates and health outcomes. Two hundred twelve studies (47%) included a control group. Outcomes were reported with effect estimates (n = 184; 41%), measures of precision (n = 274; 61%), significance tests (n = 335; 74%), sample size (n = 349; 77%), correlation coefficients (n = 71; 16%), raw data (n = 232; 51%), and parameter estimates (n = 91; 20%).

DISCUSSION

This scoping review and the related evidence map provide the most comprehensive look at the literature on high-concentration cannabis and health to date, to our knowledge. We developed this review at a time when the majority of states made cannabis available for medical purposes, and an increasing number were legalizing cannabis for recreational use. The frequency of use is increasing, raising critical questions for public health about risks associated with ready access, particularly to higher-concentration products. These questions were recognized by the Colorado General Assembly in its request to the Colorado School of Public Health. The scoping review depicts a heterogenous evidence base with important gaps regarding the health effects of high-concentration cannabis.

Concentrations Studied

There is a mismatch between the THC concentrations and types of cannabis products that are used now, and the types of cannabis products and concentrations studied in the literature identified. A 2018 survey of THC concentration in cannabis products sold in 7 states that allowed cannabis found that most products in all states contained between 15% and 30% THC.[22] From more than 70% of products sampled in Maine to more than 91% of products sampled in Colorado contained greater than 15% THC. THC concentrations have also increased over time. For example, the concentration of THC in cannabis flowers assayed in Colorado has increased from an average of 14% to 19% from 2014 through 2020.[23] Cannabis concentrate products have increased in strength from an average of 46% THC in 2014 to 68% THC in 2020.[23] The range of products continues to expand, including not only flowers but also edible products and a variety of concentrate products.[24]

Our review documents a wide range of concentrations in cannabis products that have been studied, with a median of 12% THC concentration, well below what is currently available on the market. Sixty percent of the included studies were published in the past 6 years, from 2017 to 2022. The low concentrations of THC studied likely reflect the restriction of cannabis for research purposes in the United States to that available through the National Institute for Drug Abuse (NIDA) Drug Supply Program.[25] The varieties of cannabis available to investigators through NIDA are limited in scope and lower in concentration than what people can obtain from their local dispensaries or the illegal market, and cannabis concentrates are not available to researchers.[26] Epidemiological studies can address the products in use, but, inevitably, their findings will lag behind what is happening in today's dynamic marketplace.

Exposure Assessment

The THC exposure dose, or amount of THC entering the body, depends not only on concentration in the product but also on route of administration, frequency of use, and characteristics of the individual using the product. We found a wide range of approaches to assessing exposure to cannabis products; most studies failed to capture all of the elements of cannabis use history needed to estimate exposure dose. Incomplete reporting of exposure

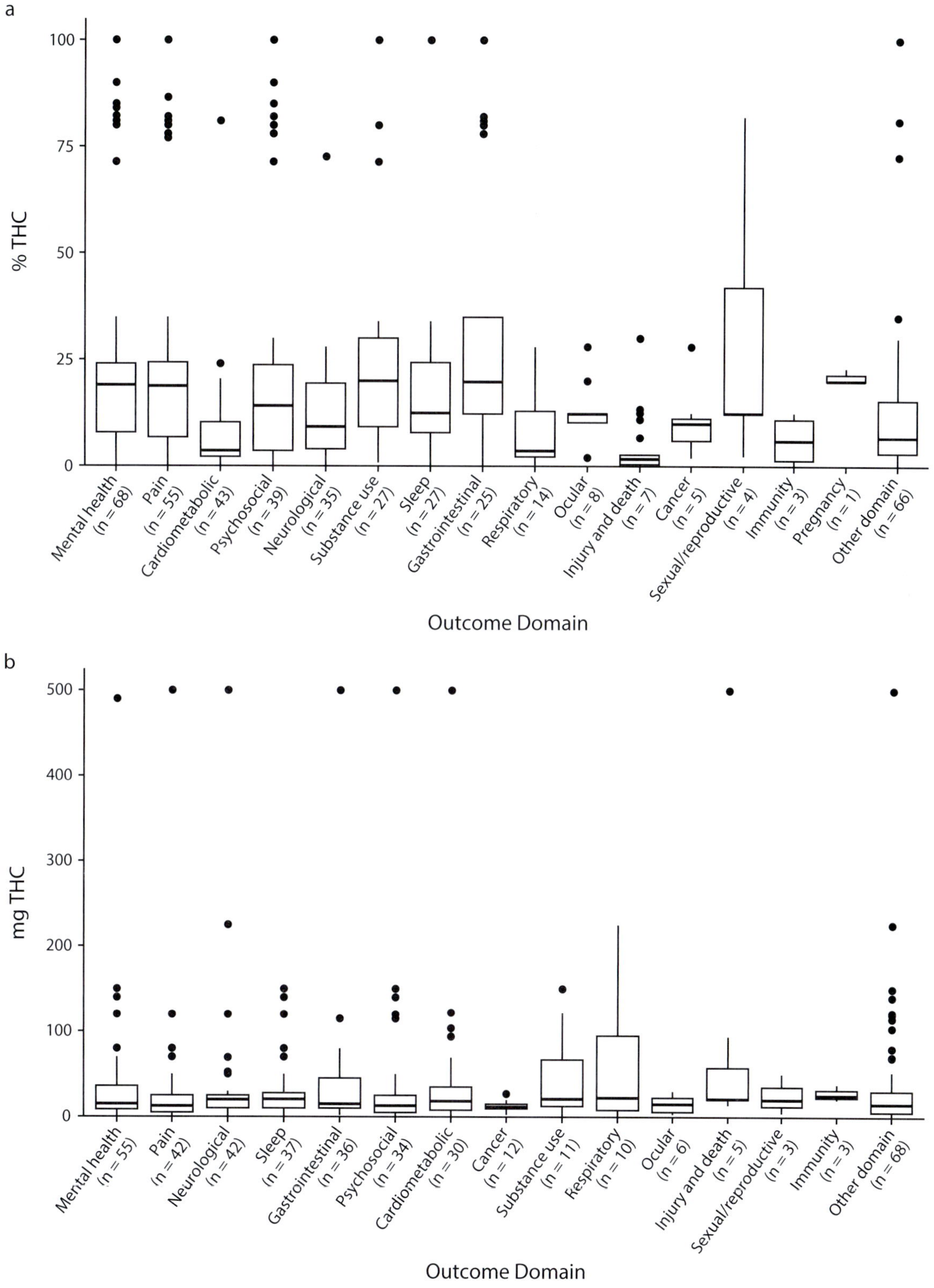

FIGURE 3— **THC Concentration Reported as Percentage of THC and Milligrams of THC by Outcome Domain in Health Effects of High-Concentration Cannabis Products: Scoping Review and Evidence Map**

Note. IQR = interquartile range; THC = tetrahydrocannabinol. Boxplot of highest reported THC concentration for concentrations reported in % THC (n = 172) or mg THC (n = 113) by outcome domain. We report data on THC concentration reported as an exact concentration (e.g., 10% THC), a range (e.g., 1–10 mg THC), a threshold (e.g., < 5% THC), or some other method of aggregation (e.g., mean % THC). THC concentration values were not standardized. The midline of the box is the median THC concentration, the top and bottom of the box are first and third quartile (Q1 and Q3), whiskers represent the Q1–1.5(IQR) and Q3 + 1.5(IQR), and points beyond the whiskers are outliers beyond this range.

characteristics makes it difficult to assess the association between exposure and likelihood of an adverse (or beneficial) health outcome.

The evidence map documents the broad scope of the exposure assessment problem, showing that THC concentration, route of administration, and frequency of use are not consistently reported, particularly in observational studies. The heterogeneity in how THC exposure was reported and measured, and in the units used also complicates evidence synthesis. The evidence map highlights a problem that needs to be addressed with urgency: attention should be given to developing systematic and standardized approaches for assessing use of cannabis products. At a minimum, studies should report exposure as THC concentration, product used, frequency of use, and route of administration, and use THC units that can be standardized. There have been significant steps in this direction, including the development of consensus standards for cannabis measurement and THC units, but these must take high-concentration exposures into account.[27,28]

Outcomes Studied

The evidence map shows that a wide array of health outcome domains, both harmful and beneficial, have been studied, as found in other recent reports.[25] For some outcomes, such as depression and anxiety, standardized instruments are available, but they are used variably. Large heterogeneity in specific outcomes studied and how they were measured hinders the possibility of conducting quantitative evidence synthesis. Bringing some homogeneity to this aspect of research on cannabis may not be feasible, given the wide range of outcomes. Within the cannabis research community, perhaps agreement could be reached on standardizing approaches to some of the most critical outcomes, using methods similar to those used to develop core outcomes sets for clinical trials.[29,30] Despite the heterogeneity of the outcome measures, the evidence map can be used to identify clusters of studies within outcomes domains that can be summarized by using narrative or visual methods.[31]

Populations Studied

Another key issue identified by our review is the range of populations studied and how well the characteristics of the study populations align with the characteristics of people who use cannabis products. Generalizability of findings is critical, but it cannot be readily gauged because we lack sufficiently specific information on the demographic characteristics of those who use different cannabis products. In addition, key populations may not be included among those studied, particularly racial and ethnic minority groups. The scoping review also revealed a major gap in use of health equity indicators. Most studies did not include any measures of income, education, poverty, employment, disability, structural racism, racial inequalities, or other indicators that would allow prespecified subgroup analysis of those who might experience high rates of adverse effects.

Limitations

To be comprehensive, our searches were designed to be sensitive rather than specific. Because of the broad search terms used, a large number of studies needed to be screened for the inclusion criteria for the scoping review. Although we used AI-assisted screening and trained graduate students to screen identified records, it is possible that relevant studies were not included. Some limitations are inherent to the nature of scoping reviews. Heterogeneity in the designs of the included studies did not allow for risk-of-bias assessment of individual studies. Such assessment could be conducted in the future if the identified studies are considered sufficient for a full systematic review. Lastly, incompleteness and inconsistencies in how studies were reported resulted in variability and gaps in data extracted.

Conclusions

This scoping review supports strong conclusions concerning the utility of the literature for characterizing risks and benefits of the current cannabis marketplace and the research approaches followed in the studies identified. The review suggests that major improvements are needed in how studies measure and report exposures and outcomes to facilitate future evidence synthesis. There is heterogeneity in approaches taken for describing products and for characterizing their use. We found serious limitations in generalizability of the studies to the current marketplace or user base.

Our scoping review and evidence map assessed all available evidence addressing the timely policy question of whether THC concentration of cannabis products should be regulated. Our review shows that high-quality evidence to address this question is scarce. However, the publicly available interactive evidence map enables researchers and other interested individuals to identify specific studies or groups of studies that address a particular question.

As the evidence base expands and improves, updating of the evidence map will provide ready access to relevant studies.

With funding from the State of Colorado, we have developed a resource that we are using to address issues raised by the Colorado General Assembly as it seeks to protect public health in the state. The evidence map is a timely resource for other entities concerned with burgeoning access to cannabis. Ideally, it will be maintained as an "evergreen" resource, tracking the expanding literature. AJPH

ABOUT THE AUTHORS

Lisa Bero and Rosa Lawrence are with the Department of General Internal Medicine, Center for Bioethics and Humanities, University of Colorado, Anschutz Medical Campus, Aurora. Jean-Pierre Oberste, Tianjing Li, Louis Leslie, and Tsz Wing Yim are with Department of Ophthalmology, University of Colorado, Anschutz Medical Campus. Thanitsara Rittiphairoj is with Department of International Health, Bloomberg School of Public Health, Johns Hopkins University, Baltimore, MD. Christi Piper is with Strauss Health Sciences Library, University of Colorado, Anschutz Medical Campus. George Sam Wang is with Department of Pediatrics, Children's Hospital Colorado, University of Colorado, Anschutz Medical Campus. Ashley Brooks-Russell is with Department of Community and Behavioral Health, Colorado School of Public Health, University of Colorado, Anschutz Medical Campus. Gregory Tung is with Department of Epidemiology, Colorado School of Public Health, University of Colorado, Anschutz Medical Campus. Jonathan M. Samet is with Office of the Dean, Colorado School of Public Health, University of Colorado, Anschutz Medical Campus.

CORRESPONDENCE

Correspondence should be sent to Lisa Bero, PhD, Professor of Medicine and Public Health, Chief Scientist, Center for Bioethics and Humanities, University of Colorado Anschutz Medical Campus, 13080 E 19th Ave, Aurora, CO 80045 (e-mail: lisa.bero@cuanschutz.edu). Reprints can be ordered at https://ajph.org by clicking the "Reprints" link.

PUBLICATION INFORMATION

Full Citation: Bero L, Lawrence R, Oberste Jean-Pierre, et al. Health effects of high-concentration cannabis products: scoping review and evidence map. *Am J Public Health*. 2023;113(12):1332–1342.

Acceptance Date: August 14, 2023.

DOI: https://doi.org/10.2105/AJPH.2023.307414

CONTRIBUTORS

L. Bero, T. Li, L. Leslie, T. Rittiphairoj, C. Piper, G. S. Wang, A. Brooks-Russell, G. Tung, and J. M. Samet drafted the protocol. R. Lawrence created the evidence map. L. Bero drafted the article. All authors contributed to data collection and substantive revision of the article.

ACKNOWLEDGMENTS

This review was funded by the State of Colorado as specified in House Bill 21-1317. The funder was not involved in the design, conduct, or publication of this paper.

We thank the scientific review committee for comments on the protocol for the scoping review and the following public health graduate students for help with screening studies and data extraction: Jamali Bilquees, Haley Burns, Hannah Craig, Madison Davenport, Austin Daw, Ashley Dehmlow, Karan Dhindsa, Emily Drewniany, Alexis Engelgau, Utibeabasi Ettah, Noah Featherman, Jackson C. Fox, Efrn Garcia, Sarah Gelinas, Andrew Jones, Colin Joseph, Deanna Kapitanec, Shania Lunna, Tenejah Mathis, Samuel Messenger, Devin E. Miller, Lydia Mudd, Natalia Rahman, Daphna Rubin, Sagun Sharma, Nicole Tabor, Kevin Wells, and Cydney Wood. We thank Neeloofar Soleimanpour and Meghan Buran for help with preparing the article.

CONFLICTS OF INTEREST

L. Bero is a paid consultant as conflict of interest advisor for Health Canada, including its cannabis committees. G. S. Wang is a paid author for UpToDate for a chapter on cannabis intoxication. A. Brooks-Russell has research funding from the Institute of Cannabis Research, Colorado State University, and serves on the Colorado Department of Public Health and Environment's Marijuana Public Health Advisory Committee.

HUMAN PARTICIPANT PROTECTION

This study did not involve human participants.

REFERENCES

1. Patrick ME, Miech RA, Kloska DD, Wagner AC, Johnston LD. Trends in marijuana vaping and edible consumption from 2015 to 2018 among adolescents in the US. *JAMA Pediatr.* 2020;174(9):900–902. https://doi.org/10.1001/jamapediatrics.2020.0175
2. Boakye E, Obisesan OH, Uddin SMI, et al. Cannabis vaping among adults in the United States: prevalence, trends, and association with high-risk behaviors and adverse respiratory conditions [erratum in *Prev Med.* 2022;159:107052]. *Prev Med.* 2021;153:106800. https://doi.org/10.1016/j.ypmed.2021.106800
3. Cannabis concentration and health risks. Seattle, WA: Washington State Prevention Research Subcommittee; 2020.
4. Retail Marijuana Public Health Advisory Committee. Monitoring health concerns related to marijuana in Colorado. Denver, CO: Colorado Department of Public Health and Environment; 2020.
5. The health and social effects of nonmedical cannabis use. Geneva, Switzerland: World Health Organization; 2016.
6. Freeman TP, Craft S, Wilson J, et al. Changes in delta-9-tetrahydrocannabinol (THC) and cannabidiol (CBD) concentrations in cannabis over time: systematic review and meta-analysis. *Addiction.* 2021;116(5):1000–1010. https://doi.org/10.1111/add.15253
7. ProCon/Encyclopedia Brittanica. Legal medical marijuana states and DC. ProCon. Available at: https://medicalmarijuana.procon.org/legal-medical-marijuana-states-and-dc. Accessed April 2, 2020.
8. National Conference of State Legislatures. Cannabis overview. May 31, 2022. Available at: https://www.ncsl.org/civil-and-criminal-justice/cannabis-overview. Accessed February 16, 2023.
9. Regulating Marijuana Concentrates. Colorado HB21-1317. ALS 313. 2021.
10. Colquhoun HL, Levac D, O'Brien KK, et al. Scoping reviews: time for clarity in definition, methods, and reporting. *J Clin Epidemiol.* 2014;67(12):1291–1294. https://doi.org/10.1016/j.jclinepi.2014.03.013
11. Arksey H, O'Malley L. Scoping studies: towards a methodological framework. *Int J Soc Res Methodol.* 2005;8(1):19–32. https://doi.org/10.1080/1364557032000119616
12. Wolffe TAM, Whaley P, Halsall C, Rooney AA, Walker VR. Systematic evidence maps as a novel tool to support evidence-based decision-making in chemicals policy and risk management. *Environ Int.* 2019;130:104871. https://doi.org/10.1016/j.envint.2019.05.065
13. Saran A, White H. Evidence and gap maps: a comparison of different approaches. *Campbell Syst Rev.* 2018;14(1):1–38. https://doi.org/10.4073/cmdp.2018.2
14. Miake-Lye IM, Hempel S, Shanman R, Shekelle PG. What is an evidence map? A systematic review of published evidence maps and their definitions, methods, and products. *Syst Rev.* 2016;5(1):28. https://doi.org/10.1186/s13643-016-0204-x
15. Pelch KE, Bolden AL, Kwiatkowski CF. Environmental chemicals and autism: a scoping review of the human and animal research. *Environ Health Perspect.* 2019;127(4):046001. https://doi.org/10.1289/EHP4386
16. Bero L, Li T, Rittiphairoj T, et al. Health effects of high-potency cannabis products: a scoping review protocol. *OSF Registries.* December 10, 2021. https://doi.org/10.17605/OSF.IO/WV7E9
17. Peters M, McInerney P, Munn Z, Tricco A, Khalil H. Scoping reviews. In: *JBI Manual for Evidence Synthesis.* Philadelphia, PA: Wolters Kluwer; 2020.
18. Scoping reviews: what they are and how you can do them. Cochrane Training. 2020. Available at: https://training.cochrane.org/resource/scoping-reviews-what-they-are-and-how-you-can-do-them. Accessed February 16, 2023.
19. Evidence Partners. Ottawa, Ontario, Canada; DistillerSR; 2021.
20. Tricco AC, Lillie E, Zarin W, et al. PRISMA extension for scoping reviews (PRISMA-ScR): checklist and explanation. *Ann Intern Med.* 2018;169(7):467–473. https://doi.org/10.7326/M18-0850

21. Clarke DE, Gonzalez M, Pereira A, Boyce-Gaudreau K, Waldman C, Demczuk L. The impact of knowledge on attitudes of emergency department staff towards patients with substance related presentations: a quantitative systematic review protocol. *JBI Evid Synth.* 2015;13(10):133–145. https://doi.org/10.11124/jbisrir-2015-2203
22. Cash MC, Cunnane K, Fan C, Romero-Sandoval EA. Mapping cannabis potency in medical and recreational programs in the United States. *PLoS One.* 2020;15(3):e0230167. https://doi.org/10.1371/journal.pone.0230167
23. University of Colorado Leeds School of Business, MPG Consulting. Regulated marijuana: market update. 2020. Available at: https://sbg.colorado.gov/sites/sbg/files/2020-Regulated-Marijuana-Market-Update-Final.pdf. Accessed February 16, 2023.
24. Spindle TR, Bonn-Miller MO, Vandrey R. Changing landscape of cannabis: novel products, formulations, and methods of administration. *Curr Opin Psychol.* 2019;30:98–102. https://doi.org/10.1016/j.copsyc.2019.04.002
25. Committee on the Health Effects of Marijuana: An Evidence Review and Research Agenda, Board on Population Health and Public Health Practice, Health and Medicine Division, National Academies of Sciences, Engineering, and Medicine. *The Health Effects of Cannabis and Cannabinoids: The Current State of Evidence and Recommendations for Research.* Washington, DC: National Academies Press; 2017. https://doi.org/10.17226/24625
26. Stith SS, Vigil JM. Federal barriers to cannabis research. *Science.* 2016;352(6290):1182. https://doi.org/10.1126/science.aaf7450
27. Lorenzetti V, Hindocha C, Petrilli K, et al. The International Cannabis Toolkit (iCannToolkit): a multidisciplinary expert consensus on minimum standards for measuring cannabis use. *Addiction.* 2022;117(6):1510–1517. https://doi.org/10.1111/add.15702
28. Freeman TP, Lorenzetti V. A standard THC unit for reporting of health research on cannabis and cannabinoids. *Lancet Psychiatry.* 2021;8(11):944–946. https://doi.org/10.1016/S2215-0366(21)00355-2
29. Williamson PR, Altman DG, Blazeby JM, et al. Developing core outcome sets for clinical trials: issues to consider. *Trials.* 2012;13(1):132. https://doi.org/10.1186/1745-6215-13-132
30. Prinsen CAC, Vohra S, Rose MR, et al. Core Outcome Measures in Effectiveness Trials (COMET) initiative: protocol for an international Delphi study to achieve consensus on how to select outcome measurement instruments for outcomes included in a "core outcome set." *Trials.* 2014;15(1):247. https://doi.org/10.1186/1745-6215-15-247
31. Campbell M, McKenzie JE, Sowden A, et al. Synthesis without meta-analysis (SWiM) in systematic reviews: reporting guideline. *BMJ.* 2020;368:l6890. https://doi.org/10.1136/bmj.l6890

Health Disparities Among Sexual and Gender Minorities With Adverse Childhood Experiences: Insights From the 2021 Behavioral Risk Factor Surveillance System Data

Marvin A. Solberg, RN, PhD, Lisa M. Blair, RN, PhD, Emma C. Schlegel, RN, PhD, MPA, and Julie A. M. J. Kurzer, RN, MSN

Objectives. To identify the prevalence of adverse childhood experiences (ACEs) among sexual or gender minorities (SGMs) and examine the impact of ACEs on their health.

Methods. We analyzed 2021 Behavioral Risk Factor Surveillance System (BRFSS) data. Respondents from Arkansas, Iowa, Mississippi, Nevada, and Wisconsin completed modules on 10 individual ACEs, sexual orientation and gender identity, and health.

Results. Among the 38 483 eligible respondents, 2329 (6.1%) identified as an SGM. SGMs reported higher ACE prevalence than did their non-SGM counterparts. ACEs partially attenuated relationships between SGMs and a higher risk for depression, cardiovascular disease, chronic kidney disease, electronic nicotine delivery system use, and cannabis use.

Conclusions. Evaluating and better understanding the ACE and health outcome relationship among SGMs should be prioritized. Targeted interventions are needed to mitigate the impact of ACE-associated sequelae in this population. (*Am J Public Health*. 2023;113(12):1343–1351. https://doi.org/10.2105/AJPH.2023.307420)

AJPH December 2023, Vol 113, No. 12

Individuals who identify as part of a sexual or gender minority (SGM) group (e.g., gay, lesbian, bisexual, queer/questioning, transgender, nonbinary, two-spirit, Indigiqueer) now constitute 7.1% of the US population, compared with 3.5% in 2010.[1] Despite an increasing SGM population, this group remains underrepresented in research. As is well documented, SGMs experience stigma, victimization, and discrimination, contributing to physical and mental health disparities.[2] Recent inclusion of sexual orientation and gender identity (SOGI) measures in population-based research has helped identify health disparities and risk factors among SGMs.[3–6] However, this limited research has relied heavily on convenience samples and analyses that lack comparison with heterosexual and cisgender individuals (i.e., individuals whose gender identity corresponds with assigned sex at birth). Such comparisons must be approached with sensitivity and contextual understanding to avoid perpetuating a deficit discourse that may contribute to further marginalization of these identity groups.

Little research has examined the association of adverse childhood experiences (ACEs) with health outcomes among SGM adults. ACEs are potentially stressful, toxic experiences that occur before age 18 years.[7,8] The ACE Questionnaire was developed to measure cumulative childhood exposures. In its current iteration, the ACE Questionnaire measures 10 different adversities grouped into 3 domains: abuse (i.e., physical, emotional, sexual), neglect (i.e., physical and emotional), and household dysfunction (i.e., domestic violence, drug abuse in the household, mental illness in the household, incarcerated household member, loss of parent).[7,8]

Population-based evidence indicates that sexual minorities are 1.4 to 3.1 times more likely to report all ACEs than are their heterosexual counterparts.[3–6] Approximately 73% to 93% of sexual minorities report at least 1 ACE,[3–6] whereas 52% reported 3 or more,[5] and 30.5% to 46% reported 4 or more.[3,4,6] Among heterosexual and cisgender persons, 60% to 74% reported at least 1 ACE,[3–6] and 15% to 23% reported 4 or more.[3,4,6] However, most of these population studies used an ACE measure that assessed only 8 types of adversity rather than 10, omitting physical and emotional neglect. Furthermore, gender minority persons were excluded from these analyses.

ACEs are strongly linked with poor physical and mental health outcomes and decreased social mobility.[7,8] Population-based studies and meta-analyses indicate that individuals reporting 4 or more ACEs have significantly higher odds of reporting chronic and behavioral health conditions than do those without ACEs.[9–11] Few population-based studies have examined this relationship among ACE-exposed SGMs. Most studies that have investigated ACEs and health outcomes among SGMs have used nonprobability convenience samples. Among the few population-based representative studies that focused on ACEs and sexual minorities, sexual minority persons were more likely to report poor physical and mental health outcomes.[3–6] For example, ACE-exposed sexual minorities had higher odds of experiencing disability, asthma, depression, 14 or more days of poor mental health in the past 30 days, and substance use disorders than their heterosexual peers.[3–6] Updated research using recent data is needed, and inclusion of gender minorities is critical for understanding how ACEs affect health outcomes among SGMs, particularly in the context of recent rises in the proportion of the national population identifying as SGM.

We addressed existing knowledge gaps by using a multistate probability sample to determine the prevalence of ACEs among SGMs and to investigate the association between ACEs and health outcomes. To understand the complex relationships at play, we adopted the socioecological model as the foundation of our study.[12] By examining the interplay between the individual level, such as SGM identity, and the relationship level, specifically ACEs, we aimed to understand their combined impact on health outcomes. Thus, the overarching purpose of this study was (1) to determine the prevalence of ACEs among SGMs, and (2) to determine the association of SGM identity and health outcomes in the United States while adjusting for ACEs.

METHODS

The Behavioral Risk Factor Surveillance System (BRFSS) is a probability-based telephone survey conducted annually in all 50 states and the US territories that is weighted to be population representative.[13] Administered by the Centers for Disease Control and Prevention (CDC), the BRFSS completes more than 400 000 interviews each wave and collects data on health risk behaviors, chronic conditions, and use of health care services.[13] Optional modules for the survey include ACE and SOGI. Data for this study are from the 2021 BRFSS surveys from Arkansas, Iowa, Mississippi, Nevada, and Wisconsin, as only respondents in these states completed both the ACE and SOGI modules.

Adverse Childhood Experiences

The ACE module comprised 13 questions that measured 10 different childhood adversities that occurred before age 18 years. Previously, the ACE module in the BRFSS examined 8 adversities; physical and emotional neglect items were added in 2019.[14] Participants indicated "yes" or "no" responses to each question. In 3 cases, 2 questions assessed different aspects of the same construct from the 10-item ACE Questionnaire; we collapsed these into a single variable for consistency with extant ACE literature. We determined a total score by summing all "yes" responses, and scores ranged from 0 to 10. In regression models, we treated ACEs as a categorical variable with 3 categories: 0, 1 to 3, and 4 or more. This enables direct comparison with extant literature.

Sexual Orientation and Gender Identity

Participants indicated their sexual orientation as "lesbian or gay," "straight, that is, not gay," "bisexual," "something else," or "I don't know the answer." We collapsed these responses into a dichotomous variable for some analyses as indicated in the results and tables (e.g., straight = 1; gay/lesbian, bisexual/other, and questioning = 2). We measured gender identity using the question "Do you consider yourself to be transgender?" Response options included "no" and multiple categories of transgender identities. Because of limited cell sizes, we collapsed all transgender categories into a single indicator (i.e., cisgender = 1; transgender = 2). We coded respondents who indicated any combination of sexual minority status (i.e., gay/lesbian, bisexual/other, or questioning) or transgender identity as SGM.

Other Measures

Demographic variables analyzed included sex assigned at birth, age, income, employment status, marital status, race, ethnicity, and highest educational level completed. We coded demographic measures categorically using the categories represented in Table 1. In the case of race, we collapsed categories other than Black and White (i.e., Asian, American Indian/Alaska Native, Pacific Islander) because of small cell sizes. We examined 6 health risk behaviors using dichotomous (yes/no) indicators: current smoking, current use of electronic nicotine delivery systems (ENDS; e.g., vapes, e-cigarettes), binge drinking, heavy alcohol consumption, current cannabis use, and past-month sedentary behavior (not participating in any physical activity). We assessed chronic health conditions using the question "Have you ever been told by a doctor, nurse, or other health professional that you have [indicator]?" We recoded and collapsed responses as appropriate to inform 7 conditions of interest in this analysis: depression, cardiovascular disease (CVD; a composite of myocardial infarction, coronary heart disease, or hypertension), chronic kidney disease (CKD), chronic obstructive pulmonary disease, cancer (other than skin), skin cancer, and diabetes. Additionally, respondents were asked to rate their current level of general physical and mental health using dichotomous indications (poor/fair or good/excellent).

Analysis

First, we extracted data from the 5 states that elected to administer both the ACE and SOGI module (Arkansas,

TABLE 1— Demographics and Descriptive Statistics: 2021 Behavioral Risk Factor Surveillance System; Arkansas, Iowa, Mississippi, Nevada, and Wisconsin

Sample Characteristics	SGM (n = 2 329), No. (%)	Total Sample (n = 38 483), No. (%)
Sexual orientation**		
Heterosexual[a]	202 (0.9)	36 154 (93.9)
Gay, lesbian, bisexual, or questioning	2 127 (91.3)	2 127 (5.5)
Gender identity		
Cisgender men	845 (35.7)	17 288 (45)
Cisgender women	1 279 (54.0)	20 889 (54.4)
Transgender persons[a,b]	246 (10.4)	246 (0.6)
Age,** y		
18–24	458 (20.8)	2 203 (5.7)
25–34	453 (19.5)	3 631 (9.4)
35–44	278 (11.9)	4 632 (12.0)
45–54	257 (11.0)	5 517 (14.3)
55–64	266 (11.4)	7 367 (19.14)
≥ 65	617 (26.5)	15 133 (39.3)
Income,** $		
< 50 000	1 107 (59.0)	14 555 (45.2)
50 000– < 100 000	503 (26.8)	10 658 (33.1)
≥ 100 000	267 (14.2)	7 009 (21.8)
Employment*		
Employed	1 118 (48.0)	19 430 (50.5)
Other[c]	1 211 (52.0)	19 053 (49.5)
Marital status**		
Married	699 (30.0)	17 851 (46.4)
Unmarried	1 630 (70.0)	20 632 (53.6)
Race**		
White	1 883 (80.9)	32 555 (86.4)
Black	164 (7.0)	3 080 (8.2)
Other[d]	282 (12.1)	2 066 (5.4)
Ethnicity**		
Hispanic	169 (7.3)	1 731 (4.5)
Non-Hispanic	2 132 (92.7)	36 466 (95.5)
Education (highest completed)**		
< high school	174 (7.5)	2 125 (5.5)
High school	726 (31.3)	10 887 (28.4)
Some college	702 (30.3)	11 316 (29.5)
College graduate	717 (30.9)	14 077 (36.7)

Note. SGM = sexual and gender minority. Percentages may not add up to 100 due to rounding.
[a]Transgender persons may identify as heterosexual (n = 202) or as belonging to a sexual orientation minority (n = 44).
[b]Includes transgender, gender nonbinary, and gender questioning.
[c]Includes respondents who identified as self-employed, retired, unemployed, disabled, or student.
[d]Includes Native American/Alaska Native, Asian, Native Hawaiian/Pacific Islander, other, and multiracial.
*P < .05; **P < .001; P values determined by using the χ^2 test.

Iowa, Mississippi, Nevada, and Wisconsin) from the BRFSS. We adjusted probability sample weights using weighting guidelines provided by the CDC.[15]

Weighting. Sample weights in nationally representative samples adjust for nonresponse, noncoverage, and oversampling of some groups (e.g., race categories) compared with the population. Sample weights enhance generalizability of probability-based surveys to allow more accurate inferences about the underlying population of interest from which the sample is drawn and are commonly used in national and other population representative research. We performed analyses and data cleaning in SAS version 9.4 (SAS Institute, Cary, NC) using the SURVEY procedure for complex sample weighting designs and adjusted sample weights.

Missingness. We included participants who were administered both optional modules (ACE, SOGI) in the analysis subpopulation. We determined missingness to be not "missing completely at random" in some cases. Therefore, we included the NOMCAR (not missing completely at random) statement in all logistic analyses. This statement includes observations with missing values in variance estimation, thus reducing the potential for missingness to bias estimates.

We calculated weighted and unweighted frequencies for all demographic and outcome variables and compared them by using the Rao–Scott χ^2 test and the standard χ^2 test, respectively. Then we created multiple logistic regression models to examine relationships between SGM status and all health conditions and behaviors while adjusting for demographic factors and ACEs, reported as adjusted odds ratios (AORs) and 95% confidence intervals (CIs). Results are statistically significant when the CI does not include 1. Finally, we conducted post hoc tests to determine whether interaction effects existed between SGMs and ACEs where relationships between SGM status and health conditions or behaviors were found. In addition, to provide a more granular examination of the data, we examined associations between SGM status, ACEs, and health conditions and behaviors, comparing (1) sexual minority men with heterosexual men (excluding women and transgender persons), (2) sexual minority women with heterosexual women (excluding men and transgender persons), and (3) transgender persons with cisgender persons (see Tables A–C, respectively, available as a supplement to the online version of this article at http://www.ajph.org).

RESULTS

Unweighted demographics by SGM status are presented in Table 1. Our sample aligns with current estimates of SGM representation.[1,16] Briefly, 6.1% of respondents to the BRFSS in the 5 states that administered both ACE and SOGI modules identified as either a sexual or gender minority or both. Only 0.6% of the sample reported being transgender. SGM persons were significantly different from the total population on all demographic variables except employment status and sex assigned at birth (Table 1). SGM people tended to be younger, with lower incomes and less education. Furthermore, they were more likely to be unmarried, Hispanic, and of a minoritized race compared with the full sample.

Likelihood

Prevalence of ACEs varied between SGM individuals and those who identified as heterosexual and cisgender (Table 2). Weighted frequencies of ACEs reveal that 84.1% of SGM persons reported at least 1 ACE and were 2.30 times more likely to report at least 1 ACE (OR = 2.30; 95% CI = 1.91, 2.77) than were heterosexual and cisgender persons (69.7%). Similarly, 51.2% of SGM persons reported experiencing 4 or more ACEs and were 3.36 times more likely to report experiencing high (4 or more) ACEs (OR = 3.36; 95% CI = 2.93, 3.86) than were heterosexual and cisgender persons (23.8%).

Analysis by SGM category (Tables A–C) revealed that, excluding transgender persons and men, lesbian, bisexual, and questioning women (n = 1281; 3.3% of sample) reported 2.57 times greater likelihood of experiencing any ACE (OR = 2.57; 95% CI = 1.98, 3.33) and were 3.38 times more likely to experience high (4 or more) ACEs (OR = 3.38; 95% CI = 2.80, 4.08) than were heterosexual women. Similarly, when excluding transgender persons and women, gay, bisexual, and questioning men (n = 846; 2.2% of sample) reported 1.97 times greater likelihood of experiencing any ACE (OR = 1.97; 95% CI = 1.48, 2.62; $P < .001$) and 3.23 times greater likelihood of experiencing high (4 or more) ACEs (OR = 3.23; 95% CI = 2.59, 4.02; $P < .001$) than were heterosexual men. Transgender persons were 1.73 times more likely to report at least 1 ACE (OR = 1.73; 95% CI = 1.06, 2.82; $P = .028$) and 2.26 times more likely to report high ACEs than were cisgender persons (OR = 2.26; 95% CI = 1.49, 3.42; $P < .001$). Wider CIs and the small number of transgender individuals in the sample (n = 246; 0.6% of total sample) indicate that this estimate may be less certain than those for sexual minority individuals.

TABLE 2— ACE Scores by SGM Status: 2021 Behavioral Risk Factor Surveillance System; Arkansas, Iowa, Mississippi, Nevada, and Wisconsin

ACE Score	SGM (n = 2329), No. (%)	Sexual Minority Women (n = 1363), Frequency (%)	Sexual Minority Men (n = 903), Frequency (%)	Gender Minority Persons (n = 168), Frequency (%)	Heterosexual Cisgender (n = 35 372), Frequency (%)
0	440 (15.8)	253 (14.8)	167 (16.8)	28 (13.9)	12 849 (30.2)
1	363 (13.4)	190 (11.8)	161 (15.4)	27 (19.8)	8 031 (21.0)
2	309 (10.3)	168 (8.4)	131 (12.8)	21 (10.6)	4 927 (14.7)
3	234 (9.2)	136 (9.7)	94 (8.4)	7 (3.7)	3 037 (9.2)
4	228 (11.4)	131 (10.8)	94 (12.8)	14 (6.7)	2 207 (7.1)
5	183 (9.3)	111 (9.7)	65 (8.5)	18 (6.8)	1 673 (5.1)
6	182 (9.1)	106 (9.3)	74 (9.3)	17 (10.8)	1 266 (4.2)
7	142 (7.3)	93 (8.3)	46 (5.8)	18 (9.9)	949 (3.0)
8	105 (6.3)	78 (8.2)	26 (3.6)	8 (6.1)	681 (2.4)
9	81 (4.5)	58 (5.6)	22 (2.8)	2 (1.2)	388 (1.4)
10	62 (3.4)	39 (3.3)	23 (3.8)	8 (10.6)	146 (0.6)

Note. ACE = adverse childhood experience; SGM = sexual and gender minority. Frequencies in this table are weighted. Percentages may not add up to 100 due to rounding.

Variations in Conditions and Behaviors

SGM persons were more than twice as likely to report depression than were with non-SGM persons, as shown in Table 3 (OR = 2.80; 95% CI = 2.78, 3.29). Similarly, SGM persons had elevated risks of CVD (OR = 1.36; 95% CI = 1.11, 1.66) and CKD (OR = 1.84; 95% CI = 1.26, 2.68). Two health behaviors were also associated with SGM status: current use of ENDS (OR = 1.80; 95% CI = 1.40, 2.32) and current use of cannabis (OR = 2.21; 95% CI = 1.60, 3.04) were more likely among SGM persons than among non-SGM persons. We found no signifi cant differences in the likelihood of diagnosis of chronic obstructive pulmonary disease, cancer, skin cancer, or diabetes based on SGM status, nor current smoking, binge drinking, heavy alcohol use, or sedentary lifestyle.

Controlling Adverse Childhood Experiences

The relationships between SGM status and all health conditions and behaviors were partially attenuated after adjusting for ACEs but remained elevated compared with non-SGM persons (Table 3). Specifically, depression diagnosis remained more than 2 times more likely among SGM than among non-SGM persons after controlling for ACEs (OR = 2.32; 95% CI = 1.97, 2.74). Similarly, current ENDS use (OR = 1.26; 95% CI = 1.21, 2.02), current cannabis use (OR = 1.96; 95% CI = 1.43, 2.68), CVD (OR = 1.32; 95% CI = 1.08, 1.61), and CKD (OR = 1.77; 95% CI = 1.21, 2.58) were modestly attenuated by controlling for ACEs. An interaction effect was observed in post hoc analysis between SGM and ACEs on CVD (P = .013; Figure 1). No interaction effect was detected on depression or CKD.

DISCUSSION

To our knowledge, this is the fourth study to examine ACE prevalence and association of health outcomes using a nationally representative sample of SGMs from the BRFSS.[3–5] Our study yielded 3 salient findings: (1) SGMs reported higher ACEs than did non-SGMs, (2) an interaction effect occurred between SGM and ACEs on CVD, and (3) ACEs attenuated the relationship between SGM status and health outcomes.

In this study we found that SGMs reported a higher rate of ACEs than did non-SGMs. Compared with their heterosexual and cisgender peers, SGMs were 2.30 times more likely to report at least 1 ACE and 3.36 times more likely to report 4 or more ACEs. Our findings correspond with previous studies conducted by Austin et al. and Tran et al.[4,5] Interestingly, compared with the results of Austin et al., nearly 14% more SGMs

AJPH December 2023, Vol 113, No. 12

TABLE 3— Prevalence and Odds of Health Conditions and Behaviors by SGM Status: 2021 Behavioral Risk Factor Surveillance System; Arkansas, Iowa, Mississippi, Nevada, and Wisconsin

Health Factor	SGM (n = 2329), %	Non-SGM (n = 36 154), %	SGM vs Non-SGM, AOR (95% CI)	ACE-Adjusted, AOR (95% CI)
Chronic disorder indicators				
Depression	44.3	19.1	2.80 (2.78, 3.29)	2.32 (1.97, 2.74)
CVD[a]	31.4	38.7	1.36 (1.11, 1.66)	1.32 (1.08, 1.61)
CKD	3.6	3.2	1.84 (1.26, 2.68)	1.77 (1.21, 2.58)
COPD	6.9	7.5	1.24 (0.90, 1.71)	1.10 (0.80, 1.51)
Cancer (other than skin)	6.3	8.3	1.22 (0.93, 1.61)	1.17 (0.89, 1.54)
Skin cancer	4.1	7.1	1.15 (0.84, 1.56)	1.17 (0.83, 1.55)
Diabetes	8.0	12.1	1.06 (0.83, 1.35)	1.02 (0.80, 1.31)
Poor/fair perceived health	19.3	16.6	1.24 (0.99, 1.57)	1.11 (0.89, 1.39)
Adverse health behaviors				
Currently smokes	19.1	16.3	1.05 (0.85, 1.29)	0.93 (0.78, 1.18)
Currently uses ENDS[b]	16.6	5.8	1.80 (1.40, 2.32)	1.26 (1.21, 2.02)
Alcohol binge drinking	22.5	16.3	1.15 (0.95, 1.40)	1.12 (0.92, 1.37)
Heavy alcohol use	7.4	6.2	1.02 (0.77, 1.36)	0.95 (0.71, 1.27)
Current cannabis use	34.4	12.5	2.21 (1.60, 3.04)	1.96 (1.43, 2.68)
Sedentary (last 30 d)	24.1	25.4	1.06 (0.88, 1.27)	1.07 (0.89, 1.28)

Note. ACE = adverse childhood experience; AOR = adjusted odds ratio; CI = confidence interval; CKD: = chronic kidney disease; COPD = chronic obstructive pulmonary disease; CVD = cardiovascular disease; ENDS = electronic nicotine delivery system; SGM = sexual and gender minority. AORs are adjusted for education, ethnicity, race, age, income, marital status, and employment. ACE-adjusted AOR adjusts for education, ethnicity, race, age, income, marital status, employment, and ACE category. All omnibus models were statistically significant, with $P < .001$ as expected with large sample sizes.

[a]CVD includes hypertension, myocardial infarction, and coronary heart disease.

[b]ENDS includes electronic cigarettes and vaping.

in our study reported at least 1 ACE (84.1% vs 73.2%), and nearly 51% more reported 4 or more ACEs (51.2% vs 30.5%).[4] Our findings on SGMs reporting at least 1 ACE aligned with the findings of Tran et al. (84.1% vs 83%). However, direct comparison is limited; we focused on 4 or more ACEs, whereas Tran et al. examined 3 or more ACEs.

Higher ACE prevalence in our study can be attributed to the increased societal recognition of SGM populations, changes to ACE module measurement, and a more inclusive definition of SGM. Over the past decade, the increased recognition of SGMs has led to a rise in the percentage of Americans identifying as such, doubling from 3.5% to 7.1%.[1] The BRFSS examined only 8 adversities until 2019, when physical and emotional neglect were added, leading to more ACEs being assessed using 2021 BRFSS data.[14] Our analytical sample included gender minorities, resulting in a larger sample size compared with previous studies.[3–5]

ACEs have alarming consequences on health and social outcomes.[9–11] Cumulative exposures to ACEs are linked to several leading causes of death in the United States, including cancer, diabetes, and heart diseases.[9–11] Furthermore, exposure to multiple ACEs is linked to decreased educational attainment, reduced occupational potential, and even premature mortality.[7,17] For example, those who report experiencing at least 6 ACEs have significantly shorter lifespans, living 20 years fewer on average.[17] This is especially concerning for SGM individuals, who face a heightened risk of ACEs and, consequently, more significant negative outcomes.[3–6]

An interaction effect between SGM status and ACEs on CVD indicates that the combination of being in an SGM and experiencing ACEs has a potent impact on CVD risk. Our findings suggest that this interaction effect may be an important mechanism underlying elevated CVD risk through stress in SGM populations. This interaction effect has important implications for the development of targeted prevention and intervention programs for SGM populations. For example, previous studies have

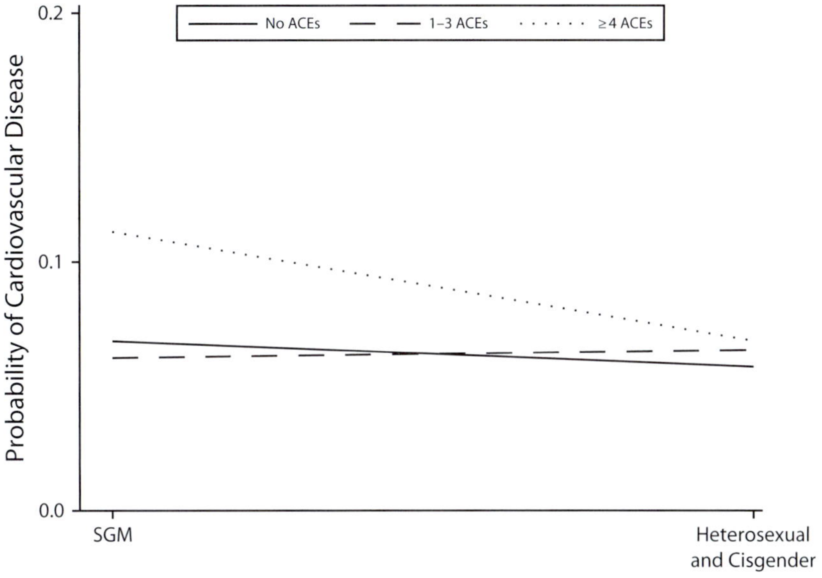

FIGURE 1— Interaction Effect for SGMs and ACEs on Cardiovascular Disease: 2021 Behavioral Risk Factor Surveillance System; Arkansas, Iowa, Mississippi, Nevada, and Wisconsin

Note. ACE = adverse childhood experiences; SGM = sexual and gender minority. The interaction effect was statistically significant ($P = .013$). Reporting ≥4 ACEs increased the probability of reporting cardiovascular disease compared with SGMs with fewer ACEs or heterosexual and cisgender persons with any ACEs.

shown that addressing ACEs through trauma-focused therapies and other interventions may reduce cardiovascular risk.[18,19] However, these interventions may need to be adapted to respond to the needs of diverse SGM populations, who may face unique barriers to accessing health care and support services.[20,21]

Furthermore, this interaction effect highlights the role intersecting identities and experiences contribute to CVD risk. Understanding intersectionality and the lived experiences of SGM persons with further marginalized identities (e.g., Black, sexual minority men living with HIV, Latina transgender women who engage in sex work) will be crucial as scholars and practitioners move toward the development of more comprehensive and inclusive approaches to meet the needs of SGM populations. Importantly, our findings align with previous studies that have shown an elevated risk of CVD among SGMs.[22,23] These studies highlight the need for further research to understand the underlying mechanisms and to develop tailored interventions to reduce CVD among SGM populations.

Although it is well established that SGM individuals experience unique health disparities, the extent to which SGM identity is directly associated with specific health outcomes is not fully understood. In our study, after controlling for demographic variables, the significant associations between being in an SGM and depression, CVD, CKD, ENDS use, and cannabis use remained significant but were partially attenuated by ACEs. Our findings were similar to those of Austin et al.: not all health outcomes were significant, and an attenuation effect was noted after controlling for ACEs.[4]

These findings highlight the importance of considering the role of other confounding, mediating, and moderating variables (e.g., resilience, coping, stigma, prejudice) when examining the relationship between SGM identity and health outcomes.[24–26] By accounting for these biopsychosocial factors, the direct impact of SGM identity on specific health outcomes can be more accurately determined. This will serve to tailor interventions that address health disparities and build on identified strengths of SGM individuals and communities, thereby shifting away from the deficit-focused lens through which this population is commonly studied.[27] The attenuation of associations between SGM identity and health outcomes highlights the intricate interplay of multiple factors that contribute to health disparities, emphasizing the need for a comprehensive, interdisciplinary approach.

Limitations

The BRFSS, a cross-sectional telephone and mobile telephone–based survey, limits causal inferences. Institutionalized adults and adults without these devices are excluded from participating. Additionally, the BRFSS is a self-report survey and is subject to recall bias and social desirability bias. These factors may influence how respondents report retrospective ACE experiences, SGM status, and health conditions and behaviors. Previous studies have highlighted that retrospective ACE reporting may yield underreporting of ACEs.[28] Furthermore, the current ACE module lacks SGM-specific adversities (e.g., homonegativity at home or school, violence).[29] Thus, the true burden of ACEs among SGMs has yet to be understood.

Although we dichotomized SGM identity in our main analyses, we examined specific SGM identities in our supplemental analyses. Future surveys must incorporate more refined data into subgroups of SGM identities and oversample these populations to fully capture the diverse and unique experiences of various subgroups in the SGM community.

Another limitation is that data highlighting SGM status may not be truly nationally representative because only 5 states (Arkansas, Iowa, Mississippi, Nevada, and Wisconsin) elect to administer both the ACE and SOGI modules. Except for Nevada, these states have relatively low proportions of their populations identifying as SGM, particularly gender minority persons who are not youths.[16,30] Furthermore, cultural differences and varying risk factors may hinder expression of SGM identity in these states. For instance, gender-affirming care bans in these states (except Nevada) could engender a climate of fear, deterring identity disclosure.[31] At the policy level, all states should elect to administer ACE and SOGI modules in future data waves to provide a more representative basis; however, such bans could pose challenges to data collection efforts.

Finally, although the inclusion of gender minority persons is a strength of this analysis, their small cell sizes pose challenges to generalizability. In particular, the supplemental analysis examining transgender compared with cisgender persons should be interpreted with caution because of the inherent risks of population representative strategies when examining small subpopulations. Including an ACE module in national, population-based studies of transgender persons would improve future research. Likewise, we recommend examining gender minority persons using a case–control matched sample strategy to prevent potential misclassification bias related to sampling strategies. This strategy has previously been employed with BRFSS data examining outcomes of racial minority transgender persons.[32]

Conclusions

The impact of ACEs on health outcomes in SGM populations is critical. Our study demonstrates that SGMs face a heightened risk for ACE exposure, which has been shown to increase their likelihood of experiencing negative health outcomes. Thus, prioritizing ACE evaluation in SGMs is crucial to understand the link with health outcomes. Additionally, future research should investigate other risk and protective factors, such as minority stressors and resilience, that may influence the ACE and health outcome relationship in SGMs. To mitigate the adverse effects of ACEs, secondary prevention interventions that are specifically tailored for SGMs are crucial. This will ensure that the unique needs of SGMs are addressed, reducing their risk for morbidity and mortality. AJPH

ABOUT THE AUTHORS

Marvin A. Solberg and Lisa M. Blair are assistant professors with the College of Nursing, Wayne State University, Detroit, MI. Emma C. Schlegel is an assistant professor with the College of Nursing, Michigan State University, East Lansing. Julie A. M. J. Kurzer is a PhD student with the College of Nursing, Wayne State University.

CORRESPONDENCE

Correspondence should be sent to Marvin A. Solberg, 5557 Cass Ave, Cohn 358, Detroit, MI 48202 (e-mail: marvin.solberg@wayne.edu). Reprints can be ordered at http://www.ajph.org by clicking the "Reprints" link.

PUBLICATION INFORMATION

Full Citation: Solberg MA, Blair LM, Schlegel EC, Kurzer JAMJ. Health disparities among sexual and gender minorities with adverse childhood experiences: insights from the 2021 Behavioral Risk Factor Surveillance System data. *Am J Public Health*. 2023;113(12):1343–1351.

Acceptance Date: August 16, 2023.

DOI: https://doi.org/10.2105/AJPH.2023.307420

CONTRIBUTORS

M. A. Solberg conceptualized the study and drafted the content. M. A. Solberg and L. M. Blair interpreted the data. L. M. Blair analyzed the data. All authors revised the content and approved the final version for publication.

ACKNOWLEDGMENTS

We would like to thank Rick Zimmerman, PhD, for reviewing our article and providing feedback.

CONFLICTS OF INTEREST

The authors have no conflicts of interest to report.

HUMAN PARTICIPANT PROTECTION

No protocol approval was required, as data were obtained from secondary sources.

REFERENCES

1. Jones JM. LGBT identification in US ticks up to 7.1%. February 17, 2022. Available at: https://news.gallup.com/poll/389792/lgbt-identification-ticks-up.aspx. Accessed September 11, 2022.
2. Meyer IH. Prejudice, social stress, and mental health in lesbian, gay, and bisexual populations: conceptual issues and research evidence. *Psychol Bull*. 2003;129(5):674–697. https://doi.org/10.1037/0033-2909.129.5.674
3. Blosnich JR, Andersen JP. Thursday's child: the role of adverse childhood experiences in explaining mental health disparities among lesbian, gay, and bisexual US adults. *Soc Psychiatry Psychiatr Epidemiol*. 2015;50(2):335–338. https://doi.org/10.1007/s00127-014-0955-4
4. Austin A, Herrick H, Proescholdbell S. Adverse childhood experiences related to poor adult health among lesbian, gay, and bisexual individuals. *Am J Public Health*. 2016;106(2):314–320. https://doi.org/10.2105/AJPH.2015.302904
5. Tran NM, Henkhaus LE, Gonzales G. Adverse childhood experiences and mental distress among US adults by sexual orientation. *JAMA Psychiatry*. 2022;79(4):377–379. https://doi.org/10.1001/jamapsychiatry.2022.0001
6. McCabe SE, Hughes TL, West BT, et al. Sexual orientation, adverse childhood experiences, and comorbid *DSM-5* substance use and mental health disorders. *J Clin Psychiatry*. 2020;81(6):20m13291. https://doi.org/10.4088/JCP.20m13291
7. Centers for Disease Control and Prevention. Fast facts: preventing adverse childhood experiences. June 29, 2023. Available at: https://www.cdc.gov/violenceprevention/aces/fastfact.html. Accessed October 6, 2023.
8. Felitti VJ, Anda RF, Nordenberg D, et al. Relationship of childhood abuse and household dysfunction to many of the leading causes of death in adults. the Adverse Childhood Experiences (ACE) Study. *Am J Prev Med*. 1998;14(4):245–258. https://doi.org/10.1016/S0749-3797(98)00017-8
9. Centers for Disease Control and Prevention. Vital signs: estimated proportion of adult health problems attributable to adverse childhood experiences and implications for prevention—25 states, 2015–2017. *MMWR Morb Mortal Wkly Rep*.

2019;68(44):999–1005. https://doi.org/10.15585/mmwr.mm6844e1

10. Bellis MA, Hughes K, Hardcastle K, et al. The impact of adverse childhood experiences on health service use across the life course using a retrospective cohort study. *J Health Serv Res Policy.* 2017;22(3):168–177. https://doi.org/10.1177/1355819617706720
11. Petruccelli K, Davis J, Berman T. Adverse childhood experiences and associated health outcomes: a systematic review and meta-analysis. *Child Abuse Negl.* 2019;97:104127. https://doi.org/10.1016/j.chiabu.2019.104127
12. Bronfenbrenner U. Ecological systems theory. In: Kazdin AE, ed. *Encyclopedia of Psychology.* Vol 3. Oxford, UK: Oxford University Press; 2000:129–133. https://doi.org/10.1037/10518-046
13. Centers for Disease Control and Prevention. About BRFSS. May 16, 2014. Available at: https://www.cdc.gov/brfss/about/index.htm. Accessed January 26, 2023.
14. Centers for Disease Control and Prevention. Behavioral Risk Factor Surveillance System ACE data. June 29, 2023. Available at: https://www.cdc.gov/violenceprevention/aces/ace-brfss.html. Accessed July 17, 2023.
15. Centers for Disease Control and Prevention. Complex sampling weights and preparing 2021 BRFSS module data for analysis. July 2022. Available at: https://www.cdc.gov/brfss/annual_data/2021/pdf/complex-sampling-weights-and-preparing-module-data-for-analysis-2021-508.pdf. Accessed October 5, 2023.
16. Conron KJ, Goldberg SK. Adult LGBT population in the United States. July 2020. Available at: https://williamsinstitute.law.ucla.edu/publications/adult-lgbt-pop-us. Accessed October 5, 2023.
17. Brown DW, Anda RF, Tiemeier H, et al. Adverse childhood experiences and the risk of premature mortality. *Am J Prev Med.* 2009;37(5):389–396. https://doi.org/10.1016/j.amepre.2009.06.021
18. Godoy LC, Frankfurter C, Cooper M, Lay C, Maunder R, Farkouh ME. Association of adverse childhood experiences with cardiovascular disease later in life: a review. *JAMA Cardiol.* 2021;6(2):228–235. https://doi.org/10.1001/jamacardio.2020.6050
19. Oral R, Ramirez M, Coohey C, et al. Adverse childhood experiences and trauma informed care: the future of health care. *Pediatr Res.* 2016;79(1-2):227–233. https://doi.org/10.1038/pr.2015.197
20. Jackson CL, Agénor M, Johnson DA, Austin SB, Kawachi I. Sexual orientation identity disparities in health behaviors, outcomes, and services use among men and women in the United States: a cross-sectional study. *BMC Public Health.* 2016;16(1):1–11. https://doi.org/10.1186/s12889-016-3467-1
21. Operario D, Gamarel KE, Grin BM, et al. Sexual minority health disparities in adult men and women in the United States: National Health and Nutrition Examination Survey, 2001–2010. *Am J Public Health.* 2015;105(10):e27–e34. https://doi.org/10.2105/AJPH.2015.302762
22. Caceres BA, Streed CG. Cardiovascular health concerns in sexual and gender minority populations. *Nat Rev Cardiol.* 2021;18(4):227–228. https://doi.org/10.1038/s41569-021-00518-3
23. Caceres BA, Streed CG, Corliss HL, et al. Assessing and addressing cardiovascular health in LGBTQ adults: a scientific statement from the American Heart Association. *Circulation.* 2020;142(19):e321–e332. https://doi.org/10.1161/CIR.0000000000000914
24. Park E, Lee J, Han J. The association between adverse childhood experiences and young adult outcomes: a scoping study. *Child Youth Serv Rev.* 2021;123:1–13. https://doi.org/10.1016/j.childyouth.2020.105916
25. Solberg MA, Peters RM, Resko SM, Templin TT. Does coping mediate the relationship between adverse childhood experiences and health outcomes in young adults? *J Child Adolesc Trauma.* 2023;16(3):615–627. https://doi.org/10.1007/s40653-023-00527-z
26. Schnarrs PW, Stone AL, Salcido R, Georgiou C, Zhou X, Nemeroff CB. The moderating effect of resilience on the relationship between adverse childhood experiences (ACEs) and quality of physical and mental health among adult sexual and gender minorities. *Behav Med.* 2020;46(3-4):366–374. https://doi.org/10.1080/08964289.2020.1727406
27. Edwards OW, Lev E, Obedin-Maliver J, et al. Our pride, our joy: an intersectional constructivist grounded theory analysis of resources that promote resilience in SGM communities. *PLoS One.* 2023;18(2):e0280787. https://doi.org/10.1371/journal.pone.0280787
28. Reuben A, Moffitt TE, Caspi A, et al. Lest we forget: comparing retrospective and prospective assessments of adverse childhood experiences in the prediction of adult health. *J Child Psychol Psychiatry.* 2016;57(10):1103–1112. https://doi.org/10.1111/jcpp.12621
29. Schnarrs PW, Stone AL, Bond MA, Salcido R, Dorri AA, Nemeroff CB. Development and psychometric properties of the sexual and gender minority adverse childhood experiences (SGM-ACEs): effect on sexual and gender minority adult mental health. *Child Abuse Negl.* 2022;127:105570. https://doi.org/10.1016/j.chiabu.2022.105570
30. Herman JL, Flores AR, O'Neill KK. How many adults and youth identify as transgender in the United States? 2022. Available at: https://williamsinstitute.law.ucla.edu/wp-content/uploads/Trans-Pop-Update-Jun-2022.pdf. Accessed October 5, 2023.
31. Human Rights Campaign. Map: attacks on gender affirming care by state. September 5, 2023. Available at: https://www.hrc.org/resources/attacks-on-gender-affirming-care-by-state-map. Accessed July 17, 2023.
32. Lett E, Asabor EN, Beltrán S, Dowshen N. Characterizing health inequities for the US transgender Hispanic population using the Behavioral Risk Factor Surveillance System. *Transgend Health.* 2021;6(5):275–283. https://doi.org/10.1089/trgh.2020.0095

Incarceration Status Among Individuals Obtaining Abortion in the United States, 2020

Marielle Kirstein, BA, Liza Fuentes, DPH, MPH, and Carolyn Sufrin, MD, PhD

Objectives. To examine the abortion frequency among incarcerated people before *Dobbs v Jackson Women's Health Organization* was decided.

Methods. We used data from the 2020 Abortion Provider Census to examine the number and distribution of facilities that provided abortions to incarcerated patients.

Results. Sixty-seven clinics across 25 states and the District of Columbia provided more than 300 abortions to incarcerated patients in 2020. Eleven of these clinics are in states that now have total or near-total abortion bans.

Public Health Implications. People in jails and prisons face many structural barriers when seeking an abortion, especially with increased state abortion restrictions and an inability to travel out of state. If they cannot obtain desired care, people may be forced to continue pregnancies in harsh conditions. To address abortion access inequities, policy and research must consider incarcerated individuals. (*Am J Public Health*. 2023;113(12):1352–1355. https://doi.org/10.2105/AJPH.2023.307411)

AJPH December 2023, Vol 113, No. 12

After the Supreme Court's decision in *Dobbs v Jackson Women's Health Organization* (*Dobbs*) eliminated federal protections for abortions in the United States, research and reporting have continued to document adverse effects on people's health and well-being.[1,2] Abortion restrictions in 15 states resulted in 66 clinics ceasing abortion services within 100 days of *Dobbs* and more than 25 000 people unable to access abortion within the first 9 months of the decision.[2,3] Still, we do not fully understand the effects of *Dobbs*, including for people in jails and prisons—who have the fewest resources to overcome barriers and categorically cannot travel out of state. Mass incarceration and maternal health outcomes are both characterized by structural racism and racial disparities, raising concerns that abortion bans will have a distinctly negative effect on incarcerated people.[4]

In the United States, 3% to 4%, or roughly 38 000, of incarcerated women are pregnant at intake based on the most recent data on admissions of women to prisons and jails.[5,6] Before *Dobbs*, the courts consistently ruled that incarcerated individuals retained their constitutional right to abortion. However, carceral institutions implemented inconsistent policies: some expressly prohibited abortion; some allowed it, albeit sometimes with restrictions out of step with state law; and others' self-pay requirements made abortion functionally inaccessible.[7] The only existing study of abortion occurrence among incarcerated individuals collected data from carceral facilities and reported 44 abortions among 1040 pregnancies.[7] We examined the incarceration status of abortion patients using data from a census of clinics providing abortion care in 2020.

METHODS

We used the Guttmacher Institute's Abortion Provider Census, which contains data from the 807 clinics providing abortion in the United States in 2020.[8] Among other items, clinics were asked the number of abortions provided in 2020 to individuals who were in prison or jail at the time they obtained care.

Using Stata version 17.0 (StataCorp LP, College Station, TX), we totaled the number of abortions of incarcerated

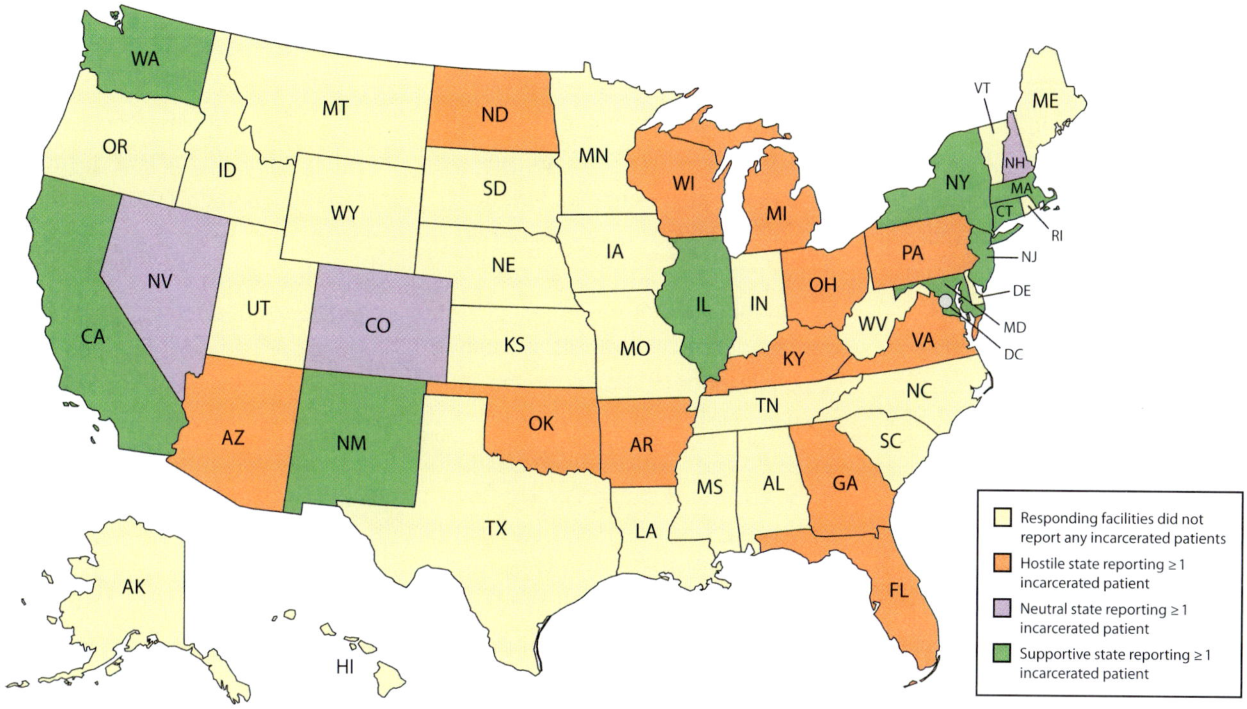

FIGURE 1— Landscape of State Abortion Policies Among Facilities Providing Abortion Care to at Least 1 Incarcerated Patient: United States, 2020

Note. Patient data reflect data from the 2020 Abortion Provider Census. Although Washington, DC, is not state based on their policies, we categorized the capital as neutral for this analysis.
Source. Nash[9] was the source for state hostility.

patients and examined geographic distribution, including state policy landscapes, where clinics reported 1 or more abortion to an incarcerated patient. We assigned states a hostile versus supportive score between positive and negative 6 based on 12 abortion protections or restrictions a state might have in effect.[9]

RESULTS

Fifty-five percent (n = 440) of clinics responded to this item. Of the 45% of clinics with missing data, 11% reported not tracking this information, and clinics with missing data accounted for 43% of clinic abortions in 2020. Of clinics that did not respond to the item, 43% were in states hostile to abortion in 2020. By comparison with other nonresponse items, 20% to 24% did not answer items about medication abortion or abortions performed after 20 weeks gestation.

Of the 440 responding clinics, 67 (15%) provided 302 abortions to people in jail or prison. The largest number of abortions any clinic reported providing to incarcerated patients was 25, and only 18 clinics reported 5 or more incarcerated patients. Most clinics (72%) serving incarcerated patients had total annual caseloads of at least 1000 patients.

Clinics were in 25 states and the District of Columbia, evenly distributed across census regions. Four states had 5 or more clinics that reported providing abortions to incarcerated patients. All clinics were in metropolitan or urban areas. Among these states, 12 were considered hostile to abortion rights in 2020 (Figure 1).[9] Notably, 52% of clinics providing at least 1 abortion to an incarcerated patient were located in a hostile state. Eleven clinics, reporting 22 abortions to incarcerated patients, were in 6 states where abortion is now banned or unavailable beyond 6 weeks gestation as of July 2023.

DISCUSSION

These data indicate that more than 300 abortions were provided to incarcerated individuals in the United States in 1 year. Given that a substantial minority of clinics were unable to, or did not, answer this question, this is almost certainly an undercount. Our data demonstrate that some incarcerated individuals obtained abortions before *Dobbs*, including in hostile states. The number of incarcerated women increased from 2020 to 2021, especially in jails,[5] and we suspect that the need for abortion services among people in jails and prisons will continue, but post-*Dobbs* restrictions will make abortion more unobtainable for many incarcerated people. Furthermore, more people, particularly Black and Brown individuals, may interact with the carceral system because of attempts to access or self-manage abortion care in restricted areas.[4]

Our results, obtained from abortion clinics, are in stark contrast to data collected from carceral facilities, which reported 11 abortions in all federal and 22 state prisons and 33 abortions in a sample of 6 jails.[7] Given that the abortion ratio in that study's jails was 18 abortions per 100 pregnancies but only 1 in prisons, it is possible that our data represent more patients in jails, particularly because more people are held in urban than rural jails and virtually all abortion clinics are in metropolitan or urban areas. Although abortion access in rural areas has long been a challenge, the geography is amplified for incarcerated people in, often rural, prisons, whose ability to travel depends on the institutions' willingness to transport them.

Twenty-two abortions in our study occurred in states where abortion is now unavailable past 6 weeks gestation. Although abortion may have been functionally unobtainable for some incarcerated individuals before *Dobbs*,[7] those in restrictive states now have no pathway for access. They cannot travel out of state, nor can they use telehealth or self-manage a medication abortion because the institution controls their means of communication. Without abortion care, incarcerated individuals are forced to continue pregnancies in custody, where they may have limited access to prenatal care, gestate in isolating and harsh conditions, be shackled during birth, and be swiftly separated from their newborns.[10] Stratified abortion access makes forced pregnancy part of people's punitive sentence. Given racial disparities in incarceration, Black, Latinx, and indigenous individuals are disproportionately harmed by this overlap between incarceration and abortion bans.

The preclusion of abortion access for incarcerated individuals in states that ban abortion raises concerns for carceral institutions' fulfillment of their constitutional requirement to provide health care.[11] Although the Federal Bureau of Prisons' policy allows abortion with Hyde Amendment restrictions, the Prison Rape Elimination Act requires providing abortion access only in accordance with state law[12]; thus in states with no exception for rape, individuals who become pregnant from rape in custody will be forced to continue a pregnancy originated in state violence.

Despite challenges clinics had responding to this item, these are foundational findings about abortion frequency for incarcerated people before *Dobbs*.

PUBLIC HEALTH IMPLICATIONS

Incarcerated individuals need, and sometimes obtain, abortions. Our study highlights how sexual and reproductive health research can and should include data about and directly from incarcerated individuals, fighting their erasure and pointing to what equitable health care might look like. Additional research examining abortion access and provision to incarcerated patients, including patient experiences seeking abortion care and what happens when they are denied care, could provide insight into the full extent of barriers to abortion care for people who are incarcerated and how policies can mitigate them.[10]

Institution- and state-level policies and access supports, such as abortion funds, should explicitly consider the needs and unique and considerable barriers to care of incarcerated individuals. Potential policy changes include eliminating the exclusion of incarcerated people from Medicaid and repealing the Hyde Amendment. Standardization and oversight of carceral medical care is necessary to ensure that carceral institutions located in states where abortion is legal have policies and practices that ensure abortion access. AJPH

ABOUT THE AUTHORS

At the time of the study, Marielle Kirstein and Liza Fuentes were with the Guttmacher Institute, New York, NY. Carolyn Sufrin is with the Department of Gynecology and Obstetrics, Johns Hopkins University School of Medicine, Baltimore, MD.

CORRESPONDENCE

Correspondence should be sent to Marielle Kirstein, Senior Research Assistant, Guttmacher Institute, 125 Maiden Ln, 7th Floor, New York, NY 10038 (e-mail: Marielle.k20@gmail.com). Reprints can be ordered at http://www.ajph.org by clicking the "Reprints" link.

PUBLICATION INFORMATION

Full Citation: Kirstein M, Fuentes L, Sufrin C. Incarceration status among individuals obtaining abortion in the United States, 2020. *Am J Public Health*. 2023;113(12):1352–1355.

Acceptance Date: July 31, 2023.

DOI: https://doi.org/10.2105/AJPH.2023.307411

CONTRIBUTORS

M. Kirstein conceptualized this work and led the analysis and writing. L. Fuentes made substantial contributions to results interpretation. L. Fuentes and C. Sufrin made substantial contributions to the writing. C. Sufrin provided expertise on sexual and reproductive health care and access for people living in carceral institutions.

ACKNOWLEDGMENTS

This article was made possible by financial support from the Guttmacher Institute.

The authors gratefully acknowledge the contributions of the data collection team, Lilian Ha, Madeleine Haas, Audrey Maynard, Rayan Sadeldin Bashir Mohamed, and Parisa Thepmankorn, as well as our Guttmacher colleagues who provided support and contributions to our product, Kelly Baden, Joerg Dreweke, Rachel Jones, Jesse Philbin, and Emma Stoskopf-Ehrlich.

CONFLICTS OF INTEREST

The authors have no conflicts of interest to report.

HUMAN PARTICIPANT PROTECTION

The Guttmacher Institute's federally registered institutional review board deemed the study exempt from review.

REFERENCES

1. Grossman D, Joffe C, Kaller S, et al. Care post-Roe: documenting cases of poor-quality care since the *Dobbs* decision. May 2023. Available at: https://www.ansirh.org/sites/default/files/2023-05/Care%20Post-Roe%20Preliminary%20Findings.pdf. Accessed October 4, 2023.
2. Society of Family Planning. #WeCount report: April 2022 to March 2023. June 15, 2023. Available at: https://societyfp.org/wp-content/uploads/2023/06/WeCountReport_6.12.23.pdf. Accessed October 4, 2023.
3. Kirstein M, Dreweke J, Jones RK, Philbin J. 100 days post-Roe: at least 66 clinics across 15 US states have stopped offering abortion care. October 6, 2022. Available at: https://www.guttmacher.org/2022/10/100-days-post-roe-least-66-clinics-across-15-us-states-have-stopped-offering-abortion-care. Accessed March 31, 2023.
4. Goodwin M. *Policing the Womb: Invisible Women and the Criminalization of Motherhood.* Cambridge, UK: Cambridge University Press; 2020. https://doi.org/10.1017/9781139343244
5. Kajstura A, Sawyer W. Women's mass incarceration: the whole pie 2023. March 1, 2023. Available at: https://www.prisonpolicy.org/reports/pie2023women.html. Accessed May 25, 2023.
6. Federal Bureau of Investigation. Crime data explorer. 2021. Available at: https://cde.ucr.cjis.gov. Accessed May 25, 2023.
7. Sufrin C, Jones RK, Beal L, Mosher WD, Bell S. Abortion access for incarcerated people: incidence of abortion and policies at US prisons and jails. *Obstet Gynecol.* 2021;138(3):330–337. https://doi.org/10.1097/AOG.0000000000004497
8. Jones RK, Kirstein M, Philbin J. Abortion incidence and service availability in the United States, 2020. *Perspect Sex Reprod Health.* 2022;54(4):128–141. https://doi.org/10.1363/psrh.12215
9. Nash E. State abortion policy landscape: from hostile to supportive. August 2019. Available at: https://www.guttmacher.org/article/2019/08/state-abortion-policy-landscape-hostile-supportive#. Accessed October 4, 2023.
10. Sufrin CB, Devon-Williamston A, Beal L, Hayes CM, Kramer C. "I mean, I didn't really have a choice of anything": how incarceration influences abortion decision-making and precludes access in the United States. *Perspect Sex Reprod Health.* 2023;55(3):165–177. https://doi.org/10.1363/psrh.12235
11. Rold WJ. Thirty years after *Estelle v. Gamble*: a legal retrospective. *J Correct Health Care.* 2008;14(1):11–20. https://doi.org/10.1177/1078345807309616
12. Prison Rape Elimination Act (PREA). Pub L No. 108–79. 34 USC, 30301(1) (2003). Available at: https://uscode.house.gov/view.xhtml?path=/prelim@title34/subtitle3/chapter303&edition=prelim. Accessed March 2, 2023.

COVID-19 Experience Reflects the Importance of Understanding the Impacts of Public Health Policies and Long COVID on Pediatric Populations

Mitchell Berger, MPH

ABOUT THE AUTHOR

Mitchell Berger is with the Department of Health and Human Services, Washington, DC.

AJPH December 2023, Vol 113, No. 12

In their well-written discussion of the 1918 influenza pandemic and the COVID-19 public health emergency more than a century later, Connolly and Golden observe how these pandemics affected children and led to lost opportunities to bolster pediatric health policy.[1] But it is important to highlight some key distinctions that can help us learn from these pivotal public health events.

First, although the authors draw some interesting parallels as to how children in Philadelphia, Pennsylvania, especially, and by implication other areas of the nation, experienced COVID-19, the "chaotic" environment existing in 1918-era Philadelphia may not have adequately represented the entire nation. Philadelphia was among the hardest hit US cities during 1918 owing in part to the stance at the time of the city's key leaders; its death rate during the pandemic exceeded that of nearly every other major US city.[2,3] Likewise, during COVID-19, differing state and local policy choices to some degree appear to have either mitigated or exacerbated COVID effects.[4]

Second, although intended at the time to curb COVID-19 transmission, such efforts as school closures, lockdowns, and social distancing had drastic effects on youth mental health, education, economic opportunities, and social development both in the United States and in lower- and middle-income nations.[5,6] Lessons learned may include being better prepared for future emergencies by considering access to technology and broadband among youths, school meals, and other needs. In addition, it is vital to fully consider, even during disasters and emergencies, public health policy impacts on vulnerable populations, local and regional contexts, and socioeconomic consequences.

Third, the authors point to the long-term health effects of the 1918 pandemic on those infected. Although it is unclear whether there were postinfection sequelae subsequent to the 1918 influenza pandemic on the scale of long COVID, we now have an obligation to ensure that pediatric, geriatric, and other vulnerable populations are not overlooked in discussions of post-COVID conditions.[7] The recent formation of the Office of Long COVID Research and Practice within the Department of Health and Human Services' Office of the Assistant Secretary for Health can help ensure that ongoing research fully reflects the needs of pediatric and other vulnerable populations.

The authors note that the 1918 influenza pandemic largely failed to change the nation's direction with respect to children's health policy. By contrast, the history of COVID-19 and its aftermath, to some degree, is still being written. Future historians, one hopes, will have good cause to judge us differently than our 1918 predecessors. AJPH

CORRESPONDENCE

Correspondence should be sent to Mitchell Berger, MPH, 5600 Fishers Ln, Rockville, MD 20857 (e-mail: mazruia@hotmail.com). Reprints can be ordered at http://www.ajph.org by clicking the "Reprints" link.

PUBLICATION INFORMATION

Full Citation: Berger M. COVID-19 experience reflects the importance of understanding the impacts of public health policies and long COVID on pediatric populations. *Am J Public Health.* 2023;113(12):1356–1357.

Acceptance Date: August 19, 2023.

DOI: https://doi.org/10.2105/AJPH.2023.307429

ACKNOWLEDGMENTS

The opinions expressed here are solely those of the author in his private capacity, have not been reviewed by others, and should not be imputed to any public or private entity.

CONFLICTS OF INTEREST

The author has no conflicts of interest to disclose.

REFERENCES

1. Connolly C, Golden J. Lessons ignored: children and pandemics. *Am J Public Health.* 2023;113(9): 985–990. https://doi.org/10.2105/AJPH.2023.307334
2. Markel H, Lipman HB, Navarro JA, et al. Nonpharmaceutical interventions implemented by US cities during the 1918–1919 influenza pandemic. *JAMA.* 2007;298(6):644–654. https://doi.org/10.1001/jama.298.6.644
3. University of Michigan Library. Philadelphia, Pennsylvania, influenza encyclopedia. Available at: https://www.influenzaarchive.org/cities/city-philadelphia.html. Accessed August 5, 2023.
4. Bollyky TJ, Castro E, Aravkin AY, et al. Assessing COVID-19 pandemic policies and behaviours and their economic and educational trade-offs across US states from Jan 1, 2020, to July 31, 2022: an observational analysis. *Lancet.* 2023;401(10385): 1341–1360. https://doi.org/10.1016/S0140-6736(23)00461-0
5. National Academies of Sciences, Engineering, and Medicine. *Addressing the Long-Term Effects of the COVID-19 Pandemic on Children and Families.* Washington, DC: National Academies Press; 2023. https://doi.org/10.17226/26809.
6. Chronic Poverty Advisory Network. Chronic poverty report 2023: pandemic poverty. Available at: https://www.chronicpovertynetwork.org. Accessed August 5, 2023.
7. Stephenson T, Allin B, Nugawela MD, et al. Long COVID (post-COVID-19 condition) in children: a modified Delphi process. *Arch Dis Child.* 2022; 107(7):674–680. https://doi.org/10.1136/archdischild-2021-323624

Connolly and Golden Respond

Cynthia Connolly, RN, PhD and Janet Golden, PhD

ABOUT THE AUTHORS

Cynthia Connolly is with the Barbara Bates Center for the Study of the History of Nursing, University of Pennsylvania School of Nursing, Philadelphia. Janet Golden (retired) was formerly with the Department of History, Rutgers University-Camden, Camden, NJ.

We appreciate the thoughtful reading of our article and the discussion of issues that, because of word count limitations, we could not address. We agree that 1918 pandemic experiences in the United States and elsewhere varied among neighborhoods, cities, and regions. The Philadelphia, Pennsylvania, experience, particularly the hosting of the mass gathering for the Liberty Loan Parade, offers a model of what not to do, and we chose it not just to highlight the impact of the pandemic but to show the baseline health context of children in the city in this era. The COVID-19 experience as it disrupted education is, as noted, both consequential and very different from the 1918 experience, when few children completed secondary education and the pandemic interrupted their work lives as well as their schooling. Finally, we fully agree that the long-term effects of COVID-19 in children as well as adults must be monitored and, where possible, addressed. AJPH

CORRESPONDENCE

Correspondence should be sent to Cynthia Connolly, RN, PhD, University of Pennsylvania School of Nursing, 2017 Clarie M. Fagin Hall, 418 Curie Blvd, Philadelphia, PA 19104-6020 (e-mail: cac1@nursing.upenn.edu). Reprints can be ordered at http://www.ajph.org by clicking the "Reprints" link.

PUBLICATION INFORMATION

Full Citation: Connolly C, Golden J. Connolly and Golden respond. *Am J Public Health.* 2023;113(12): 1357.

Acceptance Date: August 19, 2023.

DOI: https://doi.org/10.2105/AJPH.2023.307430

CONTRIBUTORS

The authors contributed equally to the writing of this letter.

CONFLICTS OF INTEREST

The authors have no conflicts of interest to declare.

THE
University of Vermont
CANCER CENTER

DIVISION OF HEMATOLOGY/ONCOLOGY, DEPARTMENT OF MEDICINE

The Department of Medicine in the Robert Larner, M.D. College of Medicine at the University of Vermont seeks a full-time, tenure-track faculty member at the Assistant Professor level. Applicants must have a Ph.D. in Population Health or an equivalent degree in related fields such as Epidemiology, Psychology, Public Health, or Data Science. Preference will be given to those with experience in global population health or dissemination and implementation science.

Description of the Position: Global population health focuses on achieving better health outcomes for vulnerable populations and communities around the world. The study and practice global health work aim to eliminate health disparities in low-resource settings around the world through research, education and collaborative intervention. Global population health emphasizes a broad, multidisciplinary approach to understanding emerging health challenges that considers the social, cultural, economic and environmental contexts that underpin health inequities. Candidates with knowledge and experience of dissemination and implementation science or data science methods are of particular interest.

We seek a researcher with skills in global population health and epidemiology to help grow the science and extramural funding of cancer and chronic disease prevention. This position will build on an existing research program focused on cervical cancer prevention in under-served populations; principally, this will include but not be limited to: 1) collaboration on a dissemination and implementation science research project in the Peruvian Amazon that aims to promote adoption of an HPV-based screen and treat model for cervical cancer screening; and 2) research on HPV vaccination in rural Vermont. The position is funded for three years, followed by partial funding for two additional years to support the time necessary to successfully compete for extramural funding. Successful applicants will be offered membership in the University of Vermont Cancer Center.

Burlington is a vibrant and accepting community located on the shores of Lake Champlain, between the Adirondack and Green Mountains. Year-round recreational opportunities including kayaking, skiing, and hiking abound. The outdoor opportunities are complemented by a lively arts and restaurant scene, safe neighborhoods, and excellent schools. Burlington is frequently cited as being one of the healthiest and best regions in the US in which to live. Burlington is a 90-minute drive from Montréal and a 3-hour drive from Boston.

The University of Vermont is especially interested in candidates who can contribute to the diversity and inclusive excellence of the academic community through their teaching, service and research, scholarship or creative arts. Applicants are required to submit a separate statement of advancing diversity and inclusive excellence.

The University of Vermont is an Equal Opportunity/Affirmative Action Employer. All qualified applicants will receive consideration for employment without regard to race, color, religion, sex, sexual orientation, gender identity, national origin, disability, protected veteran status, or any other category legally protected by federal or state law. The University encourages applications from all individuals who will contribute to the diversity and excellence of the institution.

Applicants must apply online at: www.uvmjobs.com under Position No. 00026755 with CV and cover letter. Questions about this opportunity may be directed to: Dr. Randall Holcombe, search committee Chair, via email: randall.holcombe@med.uvm.edu

Review of applications will begin immediately. Applications will be accepted until the position is filled.